It's Not About Survival, It's About Overcoming Adversity and Learning to Live Life Fully

Knowledge is Power. Tips and Resources for Avoiding Cancer and Overcoming Different Chronic Illnesses and How To Advocate For Your Health

by

Marianne Coulton

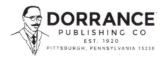
DORRANCE
PUBLISHING CO
EST. 1920
PITTSBURGH, PENNSYLVANIA 15238

The contents of this work, including, but not limited to, the accuracy of events, people, and places depicted; opinions expressed; permission to use previously published materials included; and any advice given or actions advocated are solely the responsibility of the author, who assumes all liability for said work and indemnifies the publisher against any claims stemming from publication of the work.

Dorrance Publishing Co
585 Alpha Drive
Pittsburgh, PA 15238
Visit our website at *www.dorrancebookstore.com*

ISBN: 978-1-6393-7137-2
eISBN: 978-1-6393-7948-4

*It's Not About Survival, It's About
Overcoming Adversity and Learning
to Live Life Fully
Knowledge is Power. Tips and Resources for
Avoiding Cancer and Overcoming Different
Chronic Illnesses and How To Advocate
For Your Health*

11/3/22

Marianne Coulton, May 16, 2021

KNOWLEDGE IS POWER: TIPS AND RESOURCES FOR AVOID-
ING CANCER AND OVERCOMING DIFFERENT CHRONIC
ILLNESSES AND HOW TO ADVOCATE FOR YOUR HEALTH

Preface

1   This book names many different pieces of music composed and performed by many different artists. Cancer care study results announced in January 2019 provided that listening to music you find pleasant can kill cancer cells. Additionally, if you listen to pleasant music while going through cancer treatments, it can make your treatment more effective. _NO GUARANTEE, BUT TRY IT TO SEE IF IT WORKS FOR YOU!_

2   I have spent many years listening to music to keep me calm and to comfort me when I am fearful or worried about how others treat me, or my medical treatment causes some level of discomfort and/or depression. I have done this because ever since I was young, I realized "Music is my life." When I was ten years old, I chose Cecilia as my confirmation name because I had read in the book entitled _The Lives of the Saints_ that St. Cecilia was the patron saint of music and I studied music theory then. The appendix to this book lists the music I enjoyed the most during my breast cancer treatment and afterwards while I worked hard to overcome at least five other chronic illnesses described in this book.

3   This book describes my own efforts and experiences to overcome breast cancer and to avoid any other cancer diagnoses during the twenty years following my initial breast cancer diagnosis. You can refer to an appendix of this book for tips and resources to overcome and avoid cancer and other chronic illnesses like diabetes (type II), Parkinsonism (early indication of approaching full-fledged and disabling Parkinson's disease), osteoporosis due to poor bone health, a sleep disorder, and digestive problems, dry eye and dry mouth, suggested way to restore hormones lost/damaged by cancer treatment (without putting yourself at greater risk for more cancer by taking "synthetic" hormone replacement therapy in the form of pills), and CONTROLLING

HIGH BLOOD PRESSURE TO AVOID A STROKE AND OTHER CARDIAC PROBLEMS.

4   The information in this book is for informational purposes only and is not a substitute for medical advice. This book is not meant to replace the services or advice of your medical/health care provider. No guarantees, warranties, or legal claims are made in this book. But a description of my experiences may help you (a) to explore the "root cause" of certain chronic illnesses and (b) choose a good medical/health care provider and (c) ask all the questions you should ask to inform yourself and become your STRONGEST ADVOCATE FOR YOUR HEALTH.

The names have changed in this book, except the name of my spouse, to protect the privacy of those individuals.

Acknowledgements

Many thanks to the following individuals for their review, suggested edits and comments, and information provided to enable finalization of this book for publication:

Donald J. Braverman
Lynn Shapiro
Nanette Norton
Terry Coulton
Gail-Lee McDermott
Dr. Alan Molk
Richard Toikka

Table of contents

Introduction

In April 2001, we came to sunny Florida through carefully calculated plans after the extremely sudden death of Don's brother-in-law Harold in January 2000 (we knew him well and we enjoyed his company). We were concerned about Don's sister Kathy and how she would handle the death of her husband. Because Harold's death had shaken us severely, I had argued to Don that it was time to move to Florida so Don could enjoy his life fully while he was healthy and physically able to pursue his passion—bicycling! This change was a sacrifice for me because I had worked hard to build my legal practice, which was successful, and now, I had to cut back and try to pursue a different legal practice in Florida. I felt the move was necessary for Don, who was sixty-eight years old, so he could soon begin a real retirement and we could enjoy our life together more fully. God only knew what the future would bring to him.

Our plan was that I would continue working and would be the major breadwinner. I had just turned forty-five the month we moved to Florida. I was young, active, and strong. I resolved that I would care for Don as the years went by. That was our plan. The song by Anne Murray comes to mind: "He Needed Me." But the truth is, I always needed him. By 2003 Don had saved me several times. I called him my savior even though he was not slated to die on a cross. After many years went by, when I was fearful, I said "Jesus Christ" as a prayer when I needed God's help instantly, then Don told me I only needed to call him by his first name: "Jesus." Ha! Ha! (I never meant to say the Lord's Name in vain. I needed instant relief from frightening episodes common on Florida roads.)

It is time to listen to "Jesus Christ Superstar" from the Broadway play in the early 1970s.

Part I

"The Moment": A Description of Detecting Breast Cancer Tumor Myself and Obtaining a Proper Diagnosis

After a month in our new home, I found a lump in my right breast. At the end of May 2001, it was just there. I knew in the depth of my soul that it was cancerous. It was so large and felt so hard. I did not understand where it came from. Had I been so consumed by work and our moving plans that it had grown over the months without notice? My doctor had done a breast exam in February and there was no problem. Or that is what I thought. I had the flu and a mono-like virus in March. How much had my decrease in immunity affected me? Had that allowed cancer cells to grow? Yes, it did.

I had performed at least MONTHLY self-exams of my breast over the past six months. Now in 2021 I have read there is special training available for "breast cancer self-exams" so you identify a lump in your breast before it is the size of a small ball, and it is the size of a pea! I was aware of the risks of breast cancer. The flu and virus that had sapped my energy caused me to reduce my work hours, which were normally twelve to fourteen hours a day. Now I had to reduce my working hours to six to eight hours a day. In April and after our arrival in Florida late in April, on Don's birthday, and in May while we unpacked our boxes and settled into our new home, I was still very weary. I did not understand why I was so fatigued. Now it is time to listen to "The Long and Winding Road" by the Beatles. Based on more recent reading, my problems with fatigue and immunity should have alerted me to a possible health problem. I did not catch on at that time. It is time to listen to "Danny Boy" by either John McDermott or Ronan Tynan, two of the Irish Tenors I listen to very often.

When I was dressing after a shower, I looked in the mirror

and I suddenly saw that the top of my right breast was noticeably larger than my left breast. I felt the lump. I thought the mirror must be playing tricks on me. The lump was hard, and it was large. I knew what it was; it was a tumor, and I needed to call my internist in Illinois. We had no idea where to get care in Florida; we had just arrived to live here full time thirty days earlier!

I called the internist in Illinois and told him about the lump on my right breast and made an appointment to see him when I planned to arrive in Illinois in about a week. I sat back and tried to relax and forget about it. I waited and waited, and finally, the day before my flight was scheduled to take me back to Illinois, I told Don about the lump on my right breast. I told him I had an appointment with my doctor upon my return to Illinois. I told him, "Don't worry, honey, it is probably just a cyst." Don was very worried. I assured him I was not worried. (The truth is that I was very worried, but I did not want Don to worry.) The song by Queen titled "Under Pressure" is needed now.

I had just finished unpacking the last boxes from our move and had settled into the den where I would be able to complete certain work I had begun in Illinois before our move to Florida. I had correspondence from the Florida Bar Association concerning my application to take the bar exam in a matter of weeks. I was ready for some rest and relaxation before shuttling to Evanston, Illinois, to work at my office that was staffed with my support staff and prepare for the Florida bar exam.

I was diagnosed with breast cancer in June of 2001 after I had found the lump on my right breast at the end of May 2001. My husband and I had just completed many months of planning and executing a move from our home in Evanston, Illinois, to Southeastern Florida in a beautiful, safe gated community with golf courses, tennis, and a nice social life. This was our home for the next fifteen years until our move to Delray Beach in April 2016, and then again upon our return there in May 2019. It is time to listen to "Our House" by Crosby, Stills, Nash, and Young. I gave my husband Don a bouquet of roses and a card to thank him for our new, safe home. We plan to live in our new home for the remainder of our lives. I told certain friends that my next move would be to the Jewish cemetery named "Eternal Light" near Boynton Beach Boulevard on Route 441. Don laughed even though I was serious about this and had made appropriate plans for the "move."

In 2001, I had reduced my legal practice in Illinois to prepare for our relocation to Florida. I expected to keep my Illinois office with support staff and continue to assist Illinois clients from my den in our new home and shuttle back and forth to meet with clients or perform other work when necessary. I had worked hard my entire life and never really eased up on work hours. Now was my time. I was looking forward to enjoying a more relaxing lifestyle and was prepared to form new friendships. Time to listen to Joe Cocker's song: "With a Little Help, From My Friends."

I was weary and not well before our move in April 2001. I had perked up when we started to travel to Florida via our automobile, not a simple trip for us. We had to spend several days traveling to Florida. We decided to drive to our new condominium in Florida, which I had purchased three months before our marriage in July 1998. My "child" Archie, a green wing macaw that I had begun to raise in 1990 when she was seven weeks old, could not come with us on an airplane. It is time to listen to "Truckin'" by the Grateful Dead. Archie was now eleven years old, and we were required to have a special veterinarian's certificate to take our tropical bird across state lines to her new paradise in Florida. It was great fun traveling to Florida with my child Archie. Every time we stopped at a rest stop to take a break, Archie came out of the car and greeted other tourists, including children, with a "hello" and "how are you?" Then she would throw one of her kisses. She was a big hit. Don said he could not believe how happy my child Archie made me.

Archie always came into the shower with me. She loved the special perch I had mounted in the shower stall. She spread her wings and got wet. ("Archie" is female. I had no idea what her gender was when I had bought her from the breeder in Illinois. I called her Archie because one of my favorite comic strips as a child featured a young man who had red hair that stood up at times. Archie's head had red feathers that she raised when she was excited or curious so that is why I named her Archie.) When Archie came out of the shower stall and perched above the door, I sang "Shake, Shake, Shake, SHAKE your Booty" By K.C. and the Sunshine Band. She shook her body and feathers in the shower and came out a happy bird. She loved that song.

After I detected my breast cancer tumor, in June 2001 I saw the internist who was a graduate of Northwestern University Medical School. Northwestern Memorial Hospital is one of the top hospitals in the country now. My internist reassured me the lump on my right breast might only be a cyst and he wanted me to have a mammogram. He pulled "strings" at Northwestern, and in less than a week, I was seated in the Lynn Sage Breast Clinic at Northwestern University waiting for my name to be called in a popular and extremely busy clinic. The waiting room was crowded for the morning call. Women getting routine tests looked relaxed. Many of us had never had a mammogram and were not sure what to expect. I did not think I was at risk at age forty-five. When I was forty, I never thought I needed a mammogram and thought exposure to needless X-rays was not wise at that time. Now was my time.

Many years later I urged my nieces to get mammograms in their thirties. They did not know they needed a mammogram. I told them that they did based on family medical history. (My aunt had breast cancer at some point, but I did not know until it was too late to alert me.) I do not think they knew about my cancer history, and when I urged them, they were suddenly more aware. They already should have been aware of their genetic history of cancer illness in our family and how that requires greater care to ensure a healthy and happy life. Plus, be aware of the following: Even if you do not have a genetic history of cancer in your family, it is advisable to ensure you get a regular annual screening mammogram by the time you reach age forty. If you and your doctor are not aware of family medical history, you could be overlooking important tests to identify cancer early, so you get adequate treatment. Whether you realize it or not, cancer cells could be growing that early in your life! Now it is time to listen to "Yesterday" by the Beatles.

As I waited for my mammogram, the young technician called out: "Mrs. C." I looked up for my mother, and I realized she was calling me. I was never called "Mrs. Anything" before even though I was married, because changing my name midway through my career would damage my career.

The mammogram on my left breast was no big deal, only slight discomfort. The mammogram on my right breast was nothing less than torture. I cried out in pain as the machine turned my lumpy right breast into "mashed potatoes." I cried with terrible pain. **Now, I was scared, not just worried**.

I was escorted back to the waiting room after my mammogram was completed. I felt faint. I was served orange juice. Little time passed. A nurse called for me to consult with the radiologist. A kind older woman, who was very gentle, informed me in that clinical way that I had a cancerous mass in my right breast, probably malignant. She asked why I had not had a mammogram earlier and she advised me that the tumor might have been detected earlier and I would not be in this situation now. I cried, I was numb, I was in shock. I had no idea what was about to happen or what I should do. Then, I tried to call Don and could not reach him.

See the appendix in this book about cancer screening tests. Now there are more reliable and important publications about mammograms for women than there was over twenty years ago.

After I learned the results of my mammogram, I was taken to the next room immediately for the needle core biopsy. Nine core samples were taken. Each punch of the needle machine hurt. I stayed as still as possible. I stared at the ceiling as each needle entered my right breast tissue. I did not feel like I was in my body. I must be up there in the ceiling, right? I tried to listen carefully as the doctor instructed me on how to care for my wounds. It was difficult. It was hard to feel anything. I remembered the Beatles song "Don't Let Me Down" and moved on.

Still in shock and desperately needing someone to talk to, I headed out of the clinic door. I knew I would not be able to reach Don for at least another half hour when he should finish his morning bicycle ride. I had taken the train into Chicago from Evanston and started walking back to the train station. Motion was good. I could feel something. As I walked along Michigan Avenue, I encountered a friend, a partner at a downtown law firm where I had worked six to eight years earlier. It was the gentleman who had set up the blind date when Don and I met years ago. He was aware we were both extremely interested in bicycling and invited us to dinner with him and his wonderful wife. Time to listen to "Matchmaker" from *Fiddler on the Roof* composed by John Williams. But I called him a "Yenta."

We exchanged quick hellos. He was on his way to a business meeting so there was not time for a discussion. I almost blurted out what happened to me at the breast clinic but decided Michigan Avenue was not the right place and this was not the right time. Now "Touch of Grey" by the Grateful Dead came to mind. I wondered if Cherry Garcia ice cream (not Jerry Garcia—ha, ha!) from Ben & Jerry's Ice Cream would make me feel better. I had eaten that ice cream, which has dark cherries, as a treat when I needed a break when I was studying for my law school final exams.

I walked with a purpose, and as I neared the train station, I decided to stop by the office of my first husband. He had urged me after he graduated from Georgetown Law to quit my government job as an auditor and go to law school. He said with all the difficult hours I devoted to my job as an auditor for the Department of Labor, Office of Inspector General that I could make much more as an attorney. After I passed the CPA exam on the first try, he agreed to move from Washington, DC, to Chicago to accompany me while I attended Northwestern University Law School in 1988. We were married in 1989 after his dying grandfather told him to marry me. Unfortunately, we were divorced five years later because we had a disagreement about whether I should have a child. I met Don in the same year I got divorced from my first husband and married him four years later after my child, Archie, had accepted him and I knew we could all live in the same home all the time. The Queen Song: "Love of My Life" (which I sang to a crowd of about eight hundred people in July 2019 at Mizner Park in Boca Raton, Florida) is very meaningful to me now. The crowd cheered me on after I sang the song during karaoke; women congratulated me and shook my hand, and when I was prepared to leave the stage, a gentleman helped me down the stairs and told me "You are my Golden Girl."

Ken was still a friend to me. His parents, who lived in Manhattan, still treated me like a daughter-in-law, despite our divorce. I needed someone to talk to. I walked into Ken's office, closed the door, told him my cancer news, and broke down and cried. He talked to me calmly. Ken is nothing if he is not calm. He shared the fact that his mother, my former mother-in-law, had battled breast cancer. I wondered why I had not known and then realized Ken is nothing if not discreet. He helped me calm down and he left the room while I called Don and told him the news. I was still numb. I said thank you and good-bye to Ken so he could get back to work. I headed for the train station down the street that would soon be leaving for Evanston and spotted a special purple shirt and purchased it because that was the color for the Northwestern "Wildcats" team.

The next stop was my office in Evanston. I returned calls from clients. I reviewed and signed correspondence. I made sure my secretary understood what was happening to me and that I would have times when I would not be available for her or my clients, but I would keep her up to date on my condition. She expressed great concern for my condition. Then someone from the Breast Clinic called. I listened to instructions on getting test results and worked some more. Then I went to the place where I was staying, listened to some music, and then collapsed after a long and strenuous day. That is when I said to myself: "Maybe it is time to listen to 'Bye,

Bye Miss American Pie' from 1972, composed by Don McLean at the time when Buddie Holly died in a plane crash."

I came to understand after my breast cancer diagnosis that I had ignored my child Archie's actions that should have warned me. During the early months of 2001, when Archie sat on my chest when I rested in bed, my chest had hurt. I did not know why then. Now I realized she had been sitting on my right breast when I experienced pain. My God, pets have amazing abilities. Why hadn't I paid attention to her warnings? Obviously, this was not a substitute for a proper screening mammogram. She was amazing and committed to my wellbeing. I always loved her and would continue to do so for years to come.

II. IS "SURVIVAL" ENOUGH TO STAY CALM AND RELAXED AFTER CANCER DIAGNOSIS?

They say bad news travels fast. It does. Don spoke with various family members and friends. It was not long before I was receiving good wishes and excellent support. Everyone was great and understanding. Why didn't I feel better? Was I still numb and unable to feel anything? Days and days went by. (Time to listen to "As time Goes By" played in the movie entitled *Casablanca*.) I listened to more cancer "survivor" stories than you can begin to imagine. Why don't these stories inspire me and make me feel better? What was wrong with me? I listened to Eric Clapton's song "Tears in Heaven" and cried. Was I going to die? I did not know, yet. The song made me think of my dead father. I would listen to that song almost every day during my cancer treatment to become more comfortable.

After a week went by, I confessed to Don and his sister Kathy: "If I hear one more cancer 'survivor' story, I am going to barf." I could not articulate why I felt that way. I know everyone was trying to help, to understand, to be supportive. What was wrong with me? I was drained emotionally and fatigued already. Was I tired of the stories, or was I now depressed? Who knows! I needed to get counseling. I was concerned that maybe I did not have enough fight in me to make it to the finish line. How was I going to survive? I did not yet know that I should have the goal to THRIVE, not just survive. It is time to listen to "I Will Survive" by Gloria Gaynor.

A close friend gave me a published essay to read. The essay was about a woman who had breast cancer, and yes, she died. Much of the story was interesting to me because it expressed the emotional toll on the family and living with cancer. Unfortunately, the story was more about the husband's inability to deal with the diagnosis and treatment. He left her. I cried and cried and was sure my diagnosis and treatment could chase Don away. Maybe I would not blame him. It is time to listen to "And So It Goes" by Billy Joel.

It took more time, more perspective to understand my own reaction to "survivor" stories. I could not hear the survival stories easily because it was merely anecdotal evidence. *I tend to be an "empiricist" and wanted the hard facts. So, you know, here is the definition of empiricism from The New Merriam-Webster Dictionary, the fourth publication since 1947: empiricism is defined as "the practice of relying on observation and experiment, especially in the natural sciences."* The "hard" facts would help me to evaluate and analyze my illness, my chances, and my choices. The survivor stories were touching and sometimes very poignant but not a comfort to me without more facts related to medical observation and experimentation!

Something else bothered me about survivor stories. Where were the stories about those who fought to survive and did not make it to the finish line of treatment successfully? Were there only testimonials for survivors? Was there no inspiration or comfort to be had from those who fought cancer and died? Were people ashamed to talk of a loved one or friend who had not survived? Or were they uncomfortable confronting death themselves? I wondered if I die, will anyone talk about me, or will I join the silent and forgotten dead? Finally, I realized after much agony, I had not forgotten my father who lost his battle with cancer at the end of May of 1979. Did I secretly resent him for not being tough enough to be a survivor? Was I afraid that I am not tough enough to survive? Am I suffering battle fatigue? Or is it too early for that?

Worse yet, had my cancer diagnosis led to depression that needed serious treatment so I could find a way to survive and thrive?

I have come to realize that use of the word "survival" immediately after cancer diagnosis and before surviving the necessary treatment is not good enough for improving my mental health or creating a positive attitude. I believe that creating a positive attitude is the Goal. By July of 2001, I realized, because of the course of my treatment, I could not plan to sit for the Florida bar exam. Gone was all the work I had done prior to our move to Florida to get ready to sit for the Florida bar exam. Would I ever be able to sit for the Florida bar exam? A major worry for me and contributing significantly to my depression. A song first performed by Stephen Stills during my high school days comes to mind: "Marianne." Yes, he spelled the name of the song as I spell my name. My mother who named me never allowed anyone to call me "Mary." She insisted everyone should know that I was named for the Virgin Mary _and_ her mother Anne. My mother was an "AAN." "Almost A Nun." Now it is time to listen to the prayerful song "Ave Maria."

Well, I decided I needed more than mere survival that everyone discussed when they tried to inspire me. The word "survivor" brings up images of Holocaust survivors who, against all odds, managed to hang onto life under impossible circumstances and still survive. Survival took a tremendous physical and psychological toll and left terrible scars, but they survived and left us with an image of nobility. These survivors are living reminders of horrible atrocities. I realized, on reflection, that cancer survivors fit this profile as well. But the Holocaust survivors made it their life's work to remind us all of those who did not survive. Time to listen to music from the movie entitled _Schindler's List._

Do healthcare providers or family members of cancer survivors make the same type of contribution, to remind us of the ones who fought cancer and lost their lives? Does mere "survival" fit with the positive imaging we cancer patients are instructed to pursue? I cannot attest to that. I believe the goal should go beyond mere survival and a cancer patient needs to aim to live life as fully as possible during treatment in order to create the positive attitude and avoid a deep depression so one can "THRIVE," which is needed for survival during and after cancer treatment.

III. ATTITUDE IS EVERYTHING: HOW A POSITIVE ATTITUDE DECREASES DEPRESSION AND INCREASES CHANCES OF SURVIVAL

After I had my mammogram and needle core biopsy on my right breast in June 2001, and the Pathology Report arrived; it confirmed that I had a malignant cancer tumor, stage two (for now). Later it would be stage three. As far as I know, I have never reached stage four, yet. When I received the news, I went to the bookstore to find a book to help me sort out the facts and prepare to talk to my surgeon. I chose a book that was a bit like an encyclopedia on breast cancer, and the information was helpful and comforting because the fear factor was reduced.

The book reported that a positive attitude was tremendously important in survival and suggested attending support groups to help maintain a positive attitude. About the time we moved to Florida in 2001, Don's employer wanted to keep him on the payroll to participate in certain matters in Florida. Because he remained on the employer's payroll, I was able to benefit from his employer-provided health insurance plan, and this saved us significant sums of money during and after my cancer treatment. I realized my decision to go on Don's health plan when we got married in 1998 was an excellent financial decision once we arranged for extensive chemotherapy, surgery, and radiation treatments. During 2020 I became aware that "integrative medicine" was important to obtain when you are diagnosed with cancer. Please do not wait until you reach stage-four cancer that appears to be the only integrative treatment when you search online for information about integrative medicine in Florida! See tips in the appendix for a description of integrative medicine and how it can help you survive and thrive! Integrative medicine means you have a team of medical providers to make sure you avoid depression or other significant mental and physical health problems that can contribute to the growth of cancer cells and help you identify proper treatments for your conditions and to avoid actions resulting in interference with your cancer treatment(s).

I tried my best to maintain a positive attitude once my treatment started—within several weeks after my diagnosis. I still strive to maintain a positive attitude when I am faced with other medical issues. I conduct a lot of research and reading concerning my health and wellness. Plus, I have become adept at identifying good medical providers and appealing for help from medical providers when I realize what I need and how quickly to help control my health issues. I have had great success at this over the years from 2001 through 2020, and that explains why Don calls me "Dr. C" at times, even though I am not licensed as a medical doctor ("MD"). A friend says I am an "AAD" ("Almost A Doctor"). I told everyone that I am not an MD, I am a juris doctor (JD is the degree I got when I graduated from law school.) It is time to listen to the Elton John song "Rocket Man."

Many people, including certain medical personnel think a "positive attitude" is accepting all advice at face value and never ever voicing frustration or discontent with circumstances created by my treatment. Once, I was told that "I did not have a positive attitude because I was not cooperating." It seems like my efforts to review my chart for information being withheld from me were viewed as uncooperative. That was my right, to review my chart. I am nothing if not a realist and practical. In my line of work, I am accustomed to questioning rules, regulations, advice, and choices. I have felt that sometimes during my treatment I must speak a "party line," or the words and phrases certain people want or need to hear in order to be called someone who has a "positive attitude." I cannot be passive about my treatment, and when I have been more passive (and not actively involved in decision-making), I think my treatment and mental attitude has suffered.

I cannot become a different person, just because I have cancer or because I am a survivor. I am a fighter and survivor. That is a positive attitude. The exact words or remarks I say are secondary in my opinion. Maybe it is time for an "Irish Lullaby" sung by the Irish Tenors to get ready for sleep at last. The appendix in this book contains various approaches for you to improve sleep habits so you can overcome different illnesses you may face. A friend remarked when he read this AND other portions of my work that I am "NOT JUST A SURVIVOR, I AM AN OVERCOMER." I believe, based on the past twenty-two years, he is correct. It is time for "Earth Angel" by the Penguins.

Sometimes it feels like the party line of a positive attitude is like a mantra for all the medical workers and certain other people. At times it is more than a mantra; it feels like a weapon to threaten me with certain death if I am not "positive" in the manner they require. I cannot speak positive words constantly. Who can? I am trying. Is that not good enough? The song by Queen, "Who Wants to Live Forever?" is my song of choice now.

A feeling of loss of control came with my cancer diagnosis. Events seemed to swirl around me, and I felt little opportunity to control and direct events that affected me deeply. (Well, it is important to note when I was working as an executive for the federal government, I attended a special class, and the man who administered a special personality test declared that I was a Type A [a personality type who is competitive, aggressive, and seeks control over most situations]. He said I was not just a "Type A," I was a "Flaming Type A"!)

I then had to work on giving up my demand for control some of the time to achieve certain managerial goals and objectives. The "A" is for the TYPE OF PERSONALITY not an A-hole! Time to listen to "I Go to Extremes" by Billy Joel.

When the surgeon said I needed chemotherapy, I questioned it and wondered if I really needed it prior to surgery to remove the tumor in my right breast. The surgeon explained it would reduce the size of my large tumor and could help me avoid a radical mastectomy. After giving it thought and reading about it, I agreed with his advice, to avoid a radical mastectomy, and do not regret the choice to undergo chemotherapy prior to my surgery in order to have a lumpectomy instead of a mastectomy. However, I entered the chemotherapy treatment with great trepidation for two reasons: My dad's experience when he was treated for lung cancer and my psychological and other medical issues that required certain medications that might be adversely affected by the "cocktail of drugs" administered during chemotherapy. Years later I told everyone that this surgeon saved my life. If you are on many medications, you should ensure you get good advice on "interactions" of so many medications so that you can control your health and life better.

<u>My dad's Lung Cancer Experience in 1979.</u>
In some ways I have considered myself a clone of my dad because we were close when I was growing up and shared many (not ALL) of the same thoughts and ideas and emotions. He died from the complications created by chemotherapy. Was my survival going to be influenced by his experience? Nearly twenty years after my father's death, when he was in his late fifties, Don, who was about sixty-six years of age, called me: "Mariannie." That was my father's nickname for me before his death. I quizzed Don. Had he ever met my father? What a coincidence. Maybe not. Afterall, Don was old enough to be my father. Maybe it is time to hear "C'mon Marianne" by Frankie Valli and the Four Seasons.

My father hated hospitals, and my mother nursed him at home for many months before his death. An exhausting task. He refused to go to the hospital, and I did not blame him. I have the same fear and suspicions of hospitals. (Did he learn that from my mother who had been a nurse for many years?) The day before my father died, my brother took him to the hospital. The do-not-resuscitate order was in place. I never forgot that he was in the hospital for about twenty-four hours, and then he died from the complications of chemotherapy.

His chemotherapy treatment was difficult. In the spring of 1979, before his death, my mother called and said he was dying. It was time to go home and say good-bye. I loved my dad and wanted to see him, but I feared I could not take time off from work. I spoke to my manager and then arranged to spend a long weekend at home in Omaha, Nebraska. When I flew from Washington, DC, to Omaha I had to change planes in Chicago. I tried to check in for the flight from Chicago to Omaha as early as possible. The plane must have been full, because most passengers did not de-plane in Chicago. The next thing I knew, I was bumped and got a voucher to stay overnight at the Hilton hotel. I would not ever forgive the airline for shortening my stay with my dying father. In fact, I have only flown on that airline once in the last forty-one years because I was so disappointed in the airline's "service." As soon as I arrived in Omaha the next day, I went to see my dad. He was as pale as a ghost. He was muttering and did not seem to see me. Maybe he could not focus because of the side effects from his medications. Time to listen to Paul McCartney of the Beatles sing "Eleanor Rigby."

When I looked at all the prescriptions sitting on the dresser in the bedroom where Dad was resting, Mom said he had a "difficult time with the chemotherapy." I thought that was an understatement, but it could have been a sign of "denial" that my father would soon be dead. When I said hello to Dad, he said nothing. He did not seem to know what was happening or who I was. I remembered when my father's mother was dying in May 1966, I accompanied him when he went to visit her in the hospital. I was close to my grandmother because she had helped to raise me as she lived with my parents, who worked at full-time jobs, before she had to go to the hospital. She was apparently suffering from dementia, or now I wonder if she was suffering bad side effects from medication. She looked at my father and called him the name of my father's older brother. I remember the hurt look on my father's face, and I wanted to help him. I was ten years old, and the right words did not come to mind. Here I was again. Virtually, the same scene almost thirteen years later, but the next generation. It was my turn to comfort my father again, and I still did not know what to say. Time for "Don't Let the Sun Go Down on Me" by Elton

John.

I stayed with Dad the entire weekend. We never had a real conversation. My father was now a shell, no longer the man I knew. It is time to listen to "Dance With My Father Again" by Byron Lee. I never got to say good-bye; he was too out of it. I was twenty-three and blamed the chemotherapy for taking my father away in such a painful manner. I saw his cancer treatment as a total failure. He died about a month later, on May 30, 1979. The exact same day my eighty-three-year-old grandmother had died when I was ten years old in 1966. I would always mourn them each year when Memorial Day arrived. Dad stayed home after I left, but my brother took him to the hospital near the end of May. The do-not-resuscitate order was in place, and he died. I was so miserable about his death. I buried these feelings deep within me as the years went by. The pain and the feeling that cancer (known as the "BIG C" back then) means certain death had not passed. I had awful psychological scars from this time of my life that had never healed. It is time for "Landslide" by Fleetwood MAC.

To make matters worse, I had acted two days before my father's death not to have a child at that time. I could never share this decision with my family because I thought they would disown me. After all, my mother was in the convent when my uncle introduced her to my father before she was supposed to take her final vows (she did not and left the convent to marry my father.) About five years later, she had named me after the Virgin Mary for a reason. Time to listen to the "Sargent Pepper's Lonely-Hearts Club Band" by the Beatles.

In late March of 1979, I was pregnant despite my serious, well-informed, and expensive birth control efforts, and my loving boyfriend did not want to get married. (I believe he did not want to marry me because I was not Jewish, but I had told my parents at age eighteen that I did not want to be Catholic anymore because they did not allow women to become priests.) During my high school days, I was disturbed by all the anti-abortion talk, and I thought women should have a choice because I never forgot when

I was about twelve years old that I had read about the poor women who resorted to the use of clothes hangers to end a pregnancy when they had no other safer way of ending it and that was causing more death and despair than the elimination of a fetus. I never got to share those thoughts with anyone. In 1973 the US Supreme Court arrived at critical decision called _Roe vs. Wade_, which gave women a "choice" provided they met certain requirements like having an abortion within the first three months of pregnancy. Time to listen to "Imagine" by the Beatles.

At age twenty-three, when I worked hard to meet my current living expenses and pay off my college loans (I had taken out large loans to attend a private college because my parents did not have the funds I needed), I simply could not commit to raising a child without sufficient family and friend, emotional, and/or financial support. Many women have had this experience. I did not want to bear a child that would be given up for adoption without me being able to control who the adopting parents were because there were stories floating around about the physical, emotional, and mental abuse of certain adopted children. Maybe all the people opposed to the US Supreme Court decision _Roe vs. Wade_ should act to change the rules for adoption when a woman desires to avoid the choice offered under that decision so women have "sufficient choices" when they face an unplanned/unwanted pregnancy. How could I give up a child in this type of world that almost guaranteed abuse of an adopted child? Maybe it is time to listen to the "Clancy Brothers' Irish Songs of Rebellion."

Much later, when my first husband decided he did not want to have children, we decided to get divorced. The marriage counselors we went to before our final decision always agreed with me and my description of the issues we were confronting concerning having our own children. My first husband kept wanting to go to a new counselor. Nothing changed. We eventually got a divorce. Another issue that was difficult to discuss with my family. I had been raised to believe that Catholics do not get divorced. Another choice in my life that did not yield much family support, especially now that my dad was gone. Because my first husband had been raised in New York and we had spent a lot of time there, it is time to listen to Billy Joel sing "A New York State of Mind." A favorite song that was played by the DJ at our wedding reception five years earlier.

When Don and I were ready to get married, I discussed with him whether I could have a child. He was not prepared at his age to raise more children. He had four adult children he had put through college and did not desire to make that kind of commitment in 1998. Besides, more grandchildren would be around soon enough. We got married, and I thought Don's family would become my "family."

When I got cancer in 2001 and went through a couple sessions of chemotherapy, I would go through menopause in a month and would never be able to bear children. I did not know I would be confronted with this in 1979 when my dad died or 1998 when Don and I were married. My decision in 1979, just before my Dad's death, would haunt me for much of my life, and now as I endured my cancer treatment, I had to find a way to accept the choice and move on. The song "Marianne" performed by Terry Gilkyson and The Easy Riders in the 1950s comes to mind. Like the song says most of my life I truly have been an all day and all night, person. This song was prophetic! I always was a night owl and I worked as much as possible during the day and the night. It is my nature and I have learned that my current state is partially affected by my strange sleep patterns, so I have worked hard to correct my sleep patterns without resorting to awful sleeping pills that robbed me of the ability to function properly the next day.

Developing Ways to Improve My Attitude About Life

The appendix of this book describes tips and resources for improving sleep patterns that are necessary to heal your mind and body during difficult times. You may find the tips help you avoid or recover from Covid-19 and the various strains that are passed around when people do not stay "safe" during the pandemic.

The song "Marianne" was considered a one-hit wonder in the 1950s. If you only knew how prophetic this song composed in the 1940s was. I thought of my younger sisters who I had helped to raise and had thought of them as if they were my children. But, at some point, that connection disappeared. When I attended Unity of Delray Beach, I attended services regularly and learned how to meditate and the art of patience and forgiveness. It is an "ART," NOT a "SCIENCE." One night when there was a special service that I attended, the minister taught us how to analyze our dreams. One lesson I learned was that my pets were my children; they have brought me much comfort and joy! I always have loved animals.

That same night, I also had a dream that lasted for hours now that I was no longer taking sleeping pills that "kill" your dreams! Time to listen to "Everybody Has a Dream" by Billy Joel. I dreamed about all the personal losses I had experienced in the last fifty-eight years. I had lost family members, friends, and colleagues and had faced their deaths, which I considered untimely. My God, I spent many hours in the dream recalling all fifty personal losses and awoke at 3:00 a.m. and began sobbing because my dream distressed me. Don awoke and asked me what was wrong. I explained to him that I had recalled my lifetime of losses in my lengthy dream. Then to calm myself I turned on the music on my mobile phone. I had not told "Alexa of Amazon Music" what to play but the song "He Needed Me" by Anne Murray began immediately! A sign to me that God the Father, Jesus, and the Virgin Mary were trying to help me! Now it is time to listen to "Stairway to Heaven" by Led Zeppelin.

My Reaction to Chemotherapy Treatment Based on Family History

In 2001, when chemotherapy was determined to be the treatment of choice for me, all the long-buried feelings that cancer and chemotherapy meant certain death came rushing back like a terrible flood. More than twenty years had passed since my father's death, and I was told that chemotherapy was much different in 2001. Now in 2021, there are certain better treatments available! I was told "some patients take their intravenous ("IV") treatment and then get up and go to work." I was told it was "not such a big deal." Really! It was a BIG DEAL for me! They said the side effects of the IV could be controlled. I am not sure I believed it because my father had died from the complications of chemotherapy. He had cardiac and respiratory problems that probably led to his death.

I knew I always reacted to prescription medications differently, and it took time to adjust to any new prescription and its side effects. How could I adjust to a "cocktail" of drugs which were included in the IV treatment? God only knew what could happen. My anxiety increased with each day as I waited to complete necessary heart and lung scans and blood draw tests before I could begin the chemotherapy treatment. In 2020 I discovered that the Mayo Clinic had developed an alternative to the awful chemotherapy treatment to rid yourself of cancer. This is presented in more detail in the appendix in this book.

I think certain medical providers were confused by my questions about chemotherapy and how anxious I was about the treatment. I was only forty-five years old. I think they thought for me it should not be such a big deal. At that point I had been trying for years to overcome the terrible psychological scars created when my father died when I was twenty-three years old. It is time to listen to "The Sounds of Silence" by Simon & Garfunkel.

At one point I had been hospitalized for mental health treatment, when I was about thirty-four and thirty-eight years old. I think because I could not rely on my immediate family for emotional support I suffered greatly. One doctor who diagnosed and treated me in the hospital for psychological problems said to me, "Don't worry, you are like Abraham Lincoln." It was believed Abraham Lincoln had similar mental health problems for a good portion of his life. No wonder I have admired Abraham Lincoln for my entire life. I read every book available about him when I was in college studying political science and American history. Many years later, in 2019, my brother took me to various Illinois locations, particularly a museum, Lincoln's home, and tomb in Springfield, to observe facts about Abraham Lincoln's life experiences about his home, presidency, and burial.

The doctor's statement about Abraham Lincoln was amazing to me. I was a huge follower and fan of Abraham Lincoln my entire life. When I was at a hotel in New York City, I was very afraid and worried about my mental health. My father-in-law, who resided in Manhattan, came and had dinner with me. Then early the next morning my mother-in-law, who had been informed of my concerns, came to the hotel and took me to the hospital to see the doctor, who she knew well, and she made sure that he cared for me and diagnosed me for proper treatment.

All this happened the day that Vincent Foster had died. Apparently, he killed himself and that "fact" was debated for weeks to come. That is, was it truly suicide, or had he been murdered? SCARY TO LEARN ABOUT THIS! Early in my stay in the hospital other patients on the same floor elected me to help manage our collective lives for weeks. Someone had stolen my great dark chocolate mint treats my brother and sister-in-law sent to me and I had taken prompt action to limit that kind of awful behavior, so other patients were appreciative. We prepared each day for a long walk through the city to get exercise and relax. It was an active time and a good break from long hours and days of stress that preceded my stay. Now it is time to listen to "Music for the Soul" by Thomas Moore.

This treatment helped to explain health issues I had about five years earlier without sufficient diagnosis or treatment at that time. I had a depression diagnosis and took medicines with awful side effects. I was given anti-depressants and an anti-psychotic medicine that caused terrible side effects. My first husband and I had gotten married soon after I was diagnosed with depression. I believe I had tried for years since my father's death to overcome this state of mind, but I was stressed enough most of the time that I had not overcome it. My mother unfairly blamed my fiancé for my depression diagnosis. But for years my family really did not understand me because I had left my hometown at age nineteen to pursue my college degree and had little exposure to family members for thirteen years. Now it is time to listen to "You May Be Right," by Billy Joel. It makes me laugh. <u>Laughter is the best medicine!</u>

Ways to Overcome My Health Problems, Including Fun Vacation Travel

I discovered that fun travel experiences help to relieve stress and anxiety and make you feel happier and relaxed. <u>Before my fiancé and I were married in 1989, we went on our honeymoon in Vancouver, Canada.</u> We could not take the trip after our wedding ceremony because my second year of law school would be in session. In western Canada, we hiked in the mountains and ended up hiking up from Lake Louise to a campground where we arrived before the day ended. We pitched our tent and put our food up on the "bear wire." We went to sleep. When I awoke early the next morning, I heard a bear sniffing outside our tent, and I feared what the large bear could do to possibly harm us. There was only one other camper nearby. I guess the bear thought we had food in our tent and needed food! There was snow on the ground in late August.

After the bear left the campground, we took the tent down and hiked back to our car. After our hike, we drove towards a hotel and saw the way to get on and walk on a glacier before we ate dinner at the hotel where we and many bicyclists were staying overnight.

Several years later I would have to rush home from my job at a Chicago law firm to join my first husband so we could go on a special white water rafting trip on the middle fork of the Salmon River that was in the Frank Church wilderness area in Idaho. They served gourmet meals each day of the trip, and we learned how to properly care for the environment when we bathed in the hot springs near the river. My first husband's family members were "world travelers." So, we became "international" travelers as well and traveled to London, Scotland, and Ireland while we were married. Before we were married, I had taken my mother to France, the Netherlands, and Ireland. She had never traveled abroad before, so I made all the travel arrangements for her.

During the early years of my legal practice, the law partner I worked for had a habit of contacting vacationing attorneys by cell phone even for minor matters. Not me. I warned him before I left work that there was no cell phone service in the wilderness where we went white water rafting. The food we ate was flown in daily by helicopter, and we pitched a pup tent on the side of the river every evening. Now it is time to listen to "Good-Bye to Yellow Brick Road" by Elton John.

After my diagnosis and treatment in 1993 and 1994, I experienced years in which my mental health was improved. I followed all the doctor's instructions and stayed healthy. In the spring of 1999, after I had managed my own legal practice for several years, I did not feel right. I had trouble sleeping and concentrating and was not sure what was happening to me. In my mind, this problem was tied to a terrible episode at my mother's home where I had grown up. Near the end of December in 1998, I had a snack for dinner after arriving at my mother's home after my uncle's funeral. It was December 29th, and my brother had left for Illinois right away to celebrate his wedding anniversary with my sister-in-law. My godfather, my mother's brother, was resting in the living room because he was suffering from cancer.

When I finished my snack and drank water, which had been poured for me, I suddenly felt incredibly hot and headed to the bedroom in the back of the house. I walked into my bedroom to take off the sweater I was wearing because suddenly I was hot as hell! I encountered someone I will not name in my bedroom, and she was searching through my jewelry. I asked her patiently what she was doing. She turned around, grabbed my shoulders, and threw me on the floor and then jumped on top of me and started to beat me up. I had no idea why or what was happening.

Suddenly my "attacker" who was beating me up started screaming at me that she was going to kill me and make it look like suicide and everyone would believe it! I screamed, hoping someone would appear and make her quit beating me up, abusing me, and screaming at me. Time for "Live and Let Die" by Paul McCartney. It was also time to listen to "Friend of the Devil" by the Grateful Dead. After more than an hour went by, I heard my best friend from childhood enter the room next door. She called my name, and I called to her for help. When she appeared, the attacker quit beating me and walked away probably, because she realized there was an independent third party who could be my witness in any future action I might take.

My friend entered the bedroom and asked what was wrong. I described what happened and attempted to open a window to escape the house. The window was locked, and I could not open it. I cried to my friend that my attacker had threatened to kill me. She tried to reassure me, but I was scared and in tears. Then she went to speak to my mother. My attacker came, and she started to beat me up and threaten me again. Then when my friend reentered the room, the attacker let me go. We walked out to the dining room and I began talking to my mother about what happened. As I spoke to her, my mother had her back to the kitchen.

My attacker picked up a large bottle, which was full of wine, and quickly poured the entire bottle of wine into the kitchen sink. Then she turned to my mother and told her I had drank the entire bottle of wine, which I had never touched and never had a drink other than water before she beat me up. My mother had hidden my purse and did not want me to leave. I got my suitcase and was ready to leave with my friend. My mother said I could not leave because I had too much to drink. Wrong! My attacker had lied to her. She believed my attacker, NOT ME. I quickly went to a nearby closet and found my purse. My car keys were in my jean pocket. I said to my friend, "Let us go!" Time to listen to the Queen song "Bohemian Rhapsody." Years later I sung this song for my husband a week before my birthday because certain people had frightened me, and I told my husband I was not sure whether I ever should have been born. On my birthday he gave me a card that said: "I'm Glad You Were Born."

I followed my friend to her home where I spoke to my friend and her husband for a while about what I had been through that evening. Expressing my concerns relieved some stress I was experiencing. Then, a little before midnight, I went to bed and slept for a while. At 4:00 a.m. I awoke, went to my car, waved good-bye to my friend who heard me get up, and walked out of her home. I soon began to drive back to Chicago, where I lived. Once I crossed the Missouri river in Nebraska into Iowa, I felt great relief. I had decided there was no way I would press criminal charges against my attacker for assault and battery because if the district attorney got involved, my seventy-year-old mother would be affected badly because she allowed this to happen in her home. I stopped briefly to buy gas and breakfast and spent eight hours driving home. It is time for "Let it Be" by the Beatles.

I got home by noon and was very tired because I had only a few hours of sleep before the lengthy drive to my home. I fell asleep in bed and suddenly realized that I felt I had been drugged by my attacker when I drank the water she poured in a glass for me at my mother's home. She must have put something in the water I drank that made me unable to fight back and resulted in my severe feeling of heat during a very cold winter evening in Nebraska. Was it a date rape drug? Women at a place we went to in the evening for special music picked up drinks and took them to the ladies' room with them. Why? Because they feared a man in the bar would add a "date rape" drug to their drink while they were away from their seat, and that would hamper their ability to stay safe and not experience attempted rape! When I arrived home, I told Don what had happened at my mother's home and took my parrot Archie to bed with me. She comforted me, and I fell asleep. Now it was time to listen to "Piano Man" by Billy Joel.

Later I called my psychiatrist, made an appointment, and went later in the week to him for counseling due to this horrible episode. (I was disturbed later when we lived in Florida that the psychiatrists did not counsel you. They just drugged you. They never ordered blood tests to ensure the medications were not affecting my liver or kidneys. My internist had to figure that out.) The psychiatrist in Illinois agreed with me that I should not return to my childhood home, and he kept counseling me for many weeks while I tried to recover from the horrible episode described above. Don, the love of my life, always regretted that he was not with me when I drove home for my uncle's funeral because of the terrible fear and anguish I experienced at my childhood home. It is time to listen to "Hey Jude" by the Beatles (a song I had enjoyed immensely since I was twelve years old!).

Many years later, I realized this episode had caused post-traumatic stress disorder (PTSD) and a side effect of that condition was cancer. Within about two and a half years after the episode, I was diagnosed with breast cancer! Based on recent reading, I now believe the episode resulting in PTSD had probably been a major contributor (not the only one) to the cancer I had. Now it is time for "Rocket Man" by Elton John.

My psychiatrist counseled me regularly for months after my attacker's threats to end my life and changed the dosage of certain medications. I continued to manage my law practice but became depressed because I constantly feared I could be attacked if I went home again, and therefore, I had no contact with my immediate family members, and I was unable to sleep well. When I told the doctor how I felt, he then suggested that I go to the hospital and get electro convulsive therapy ("ECT") to recover from depression more quickly, and naturally. This would give me a remedy for my depression and sleep disorder without all the awful side effects encountered with the Big Pharma medicines that only treated the "effects," NOT ROOT CAUSES (and caused serious problems if one did not take care!). I went into the hospital, and the patients I dined with could not believe I was depressed because I was relaxed and happy now that I was being freed from the awful medicines. The next morning, I received the ECT treatment. Don came and took me home. I felt like a new person! My child Archie snuggled up to me and we had a good day. Then I performed my yoga poses for relaxation purposes and prepared to return to work, because now

I finally felt well. In 2020 an oncologist I consulted about cancer concerns told me he believed getting ECT for depression was much better than taking anti-depressants when you experienced depression due to cancer concerns, and he expressed how "integrative medicine" can help you.

In 2018, due to traumatic injury caused by others who lived near my home in Florida, I had lymphedema so bad for the first time in seventeen years following surgery, chemotherapy, and radiation treatments, because I had one-third of my lymph nodes removed during my lumpectomy for breast cancer in 2001. I had very high blood pressure and excessive pain, and then I was taken to the hospital emergency room where they scanned my right arm to be sure I did not have a blood clot. Because my blood pressure was high, I became very worried. I called my sister, who was an agent named in my healthcare power of attorney. She was concerned about my health and flew down to Florida from her home in Omaha just before Thanksgiving that year. Don drove us the next day to see a lymphedema treatment expert for treatment of my condition. That night, on my sleep sofa in my living room, my sister helped me perform treatment the specialist had taught me to perform twice a day.

That evening, my sister found my six-page journal entitled "It Is Not About Survival" (not this book, yet) and read it and apparently became concerned about me. I got up and started putting up my Christmas lights for the first time in years. My sister had read the article about my cancer experiences and chemotherapy treatment and the advance healthcare directive that forbade any agent of mine to decide I should have chemotherapy if I got cancer again because I thought that treatment could now kill me.

Cancer had become a concern when I got this sudden onset of lymphedema so many years after my lumpectomy surgery. I had already cut my life back by half prior to getting the lymphedema in my right arm due to many chronic illnesses I experienced after my chemotherapy and during the period I was on ten different medicines that caused too many awful side effects. I thought to myself: "Am I to have no life now?"

My sister was upset that I might die of cancer, like our father, and is too distracted to maintain our relationship. But I have maintained a relationship with her children and grandchildren. I am their aunt and great-aunt. When I visited my niece and her boys in June 2019, we had great fun, and I told my niece there is a reason I am called a "great-aunt" by my grandnephews. I believe she agreed! Time to listen to the "Impossible Dream," which is from *Man of La Mancha* and has been performed by numerous artists for years after its composition in the 1960s.

If you must deal with the effects of post-traumatic stress disorder ("PTSD") and it causes serious lymphedema pain and sleep disorder, you can identify treatment options and seek care at the Cleveland Clinic of Florida.

It is possible to have surgery in the early stages of lymphedema to heal yourself more quickly. However, I did not go to the Cleveland Clinic doctors, and the healthcare providers who "treated" me did not suggest I seek surgery for healing quicker. I did not read about this until more than a year after I had gotten lymphedema. During early 2021, I got a lot of rest and drastically improved my sleep habits. I also found extra-strength liquid turmeric, which reduces inflammation in your body. The liquid form instead of powder form could be absorbed in my body more easily. After taking double doses of liquid turmeric (with special ingredients that increased absorption), my swollen right arm that had been constantly painful for two and a half years and deprived me of much needed sleep, FINALLY HEALED. Additionally, my escalated blood pressure had returned to normal readings on a daily basis! INFLAMMATION IN YOUR BODY CONTRIBUTES TO CARDIAC PROBLEMS and CAN CONTRIBUTE TO DIABETES PROBLEMS AS WELL! Thus, it is critical to take action to decrease inflammation in your body when you experience such health problems.

In 2019, when I went to Omaha to attend my forty-fifth high school reunion, I stopped at the assisted living facility where my mother was living because she had not been able to be rehabilitated properly after she fell and broke her leg. She was in a wheelchair, and almost completely deaf. I had a hearing problem for fifty-five years due to an ear infection when I was seven years old. Then by January 2019, I had a cochlear implant and special receiver that allowed me to hear more than I had been able to hear for most of my life. My improved hearing had many significant health benefits discussed in the appendix to this book that helped me return to work after years of health problems causing my disability.

When my brother told my mother "This is Marianne," she replied that "Marianne is not blond." I told her I was and showed her old pictures and new ones that showed my face and body was the same. I had become a blonde about five years earlier because when I grew my hair back after my cancer treatment, it was white even though I was less than fifty years old. Coloring my hair the original color of black led to constant, weekly hair dye touch ups because of significant problems with white roots. That problem was fixed when I became blond. My mother refused to acknowledge it was me for the first two days I visited her. Then on day three, I arrived wearing a name tag from my high school reunion. My mother, like me, believed things when they are in writing and finally acknowledged I was Marianne. Time to listen to the song "Feelings" by Morris Albert.

IV. CANCER AND CHEMOTHERAPY AND HOW TO SURVIVE AND THRIVE

In 2001 I was worried about the side effects of chemotherapy. I asked myself whether I could survive the treatment and wondered if it would be like my father had experienced because he died from the complications of chemotherapy. I was told chemotherapy in 2001 was different than it was in 1979 when my father was treated. I was told cancer patients like me take chemotherapy all the time and it is not a problem. How were they so sure? Were other cancer patients practicing law and risking their legal practice? Did they have extreme stress and anxiety caused by lack of support from their immediate family? My immediate family had no idea what was happening to me. Don, my husband, was my family. So was Archie, the green wing Macaw who was my "child." That was it. With great fear and trepidation, I took my first treatment in early July and wondered if I would go mad and be institutionalized. To hell with "surviving cancer." Would I survive the treatment? I eventually did, but it took more than six years to recover from certain awful chemotherapy side effects that led to "foggy brain" and impacted my legal career severely. Time to listen to "Take a Walk on the Wild Side" by Lou Reed.

I received most cancer treatments in Florida before and after my surgery. When I went for treatment, a nurse would call for me as Mrs. C. I would stand up and calmly say, "No, I am Ms. C." The patients in the waiting room, especially the males, would groan loudly. I had been a strong feminist since high school, which I think certain family members hated, especially the males. I did not change my name when I got married because it would have created serious problems with my career. I had read Ms. Magazine with relish when I was young and had learned that it could be a problem when you got married well after the beginning of your career because past contacts would not know who you were. I appreciated Gloria Steinem's advice about this, and now I was faced with hate. Were there no feminists in Florida with proper education? I wondered about this for more than fifteen years. I had never faced this in Chicago. Time to listen to "Life Is a Beach" by the Capitol Steps group.

In mid-July 2001, I awoke and started to brush my hair. Gobs of my hair came out, and I quickly grabbed almost all my hair and threw it in a nearby trash can. What could I do? I quickly called my sister-in-law. She told me she knew what to do and she picked me up and drove me to Sample Road in Fort Lauderdale, Florida, where there was a shop that specialized in assisting cancer patients who lost their hair due to chemotherapy. I got my head shaved and picked out a wig to wear and some hats to wear when it became too hot to wear the wig. Time to listen to "I Feel the Earth Move Under My Feet" by Carole King.

My sister-in-law spotted a T-shirt with a picture of a green-winged macaw just like my child Archie. She bought it and gave it to me. When I got home, I put it on, and Archie blew me a kiss. I returned the kiss. Later, Archie and I looked out the bedroom window at the Sunny South golf course outside my home. A long necked and long-legged bird was staring at us. It was a blue heron. Archie said, "Look!" We waved at the beautiful bird and laughed. This would be a habitual treat each evening during the summer. Now it is time to listen to "Crocodile Rock" by Elton John.

I went through six chemotherapy treatments that summer before my surgery for breast cancer. I suffered through a lot of side effects. Certain side effects were "controlled" by more prescription medicines. I was extremely fatigued and had great difficulty concentrating due to the medications. I designed my days to work as hard as possible all morning. By early afternoon I became so tired I could not accomplish my work and craved sleep. I averaged fourteen to sixteen hours of sleep, not work, each day. I was still numb. I did not enjoy talking on the telephone. People called and expressed great interest in learning about my health and my experiences. I thought it was a boring topic. I had to numb myself to get through the day. Talking about what was happening did not really help; my anxiety level increased, so I avoided the topic and the telephone. Now it is time to listen to "Dream On" by Aerosmith.

By the third treatment in August, I had gone through menopause completely and had to accept my fate that I would never have a child of my own. I felt like a prisoner in my body. It was hot outside. I found that my ability to handle the heat had changed. I could not walk long. I could not breathe the hot air. I quit swimming because when I put my face in the tepid water, it felt like my lungs might explode. I quit yoga sessions because my joints and muscles hurt from the stretches. So, what could I do? I discovered Twinkies on sale when we went to the grocery store, and I bought them. Twinkies were my treat of choice before my daily afternoon nap. I watched the needle on the scale daily as it moved up. I was retaining water and Twinkies! Now I wonder if all that sugar increased the growth of cancer cells. I think so now. I did not know it at the time, and none of my health care providers had warned me to avoid consuming sugar. I am advising you to avoid consuming lots of sugar while trying to get treated for cancer. I got comfort and joy from those treats but not from the results discovered after my breast cancer surgery that I had cancerous lymph nodes in the right side of my body. Now it is time for "Helpless" by Simon & Garfunkel.

Then September 2001 arrived. I got out of bed one morning and headed to the kitchen for a glass of juice or water. I stepped on the carpet in the dining room, and my feet were soaked with the standing water. How did this happen? There was a giant pool of water in the dining room, the hallway, and the kitchen. I quickly figured out the valve for the washer and the rubber hose had burst and a lot of water poured out into our condo. Oh my God, another big problem to cope with while I was being treated for cancer.

We called our insurance agent, who told us which contractor to call for help. He came quickly and evaluated the scene. He told us everyone should use stainless steel hoses, not rubber ones, on a washer to prevent leaks like we had, and if you have the rubber hoses, they should be replaced as frequently as possible. We replaced them with stainless steel hoses because they last much longer than the rubber hoses.

I spent time mopping up all the water and trying to make sure there was no moisture left in the apartment. Because of the heat and humidity at that time of year, mold and mildew had to be growing quickly. We knew by late September we would be leaving for my surgery just north of Chicago. We were told the wall separating the kitchen and dining room was full of mold and mildew and so were the bottom kitchen cabinets. I arranged to empty them before we left. When we got ready to leave, we handed the contractor our keys, he moved the equipment and new floor tiles inside because we wanted to avoid the inconvenience of living in our home while the contractor performed the work over a three-week period, and we left for the airport. Now it is time for "Leaving on a Jet Plane" by Peter, Paul, and Mary.

How the 9/11 Atrocity Affected Us

I awoke one morning on September 11, 2001, with high anxiety because I had to survive my last chemotherapy treatment before my surgery, which was scheduled for early October in Evanston, Illinois, just north of Chicago. I had barely gotten out of bed from one of my ten- to twelve-hour sleeping marathons. The telephone rang. It was an annoying solicitation. I hung up. My head ached, probably because of the medication I was taking and maybe because I had gotten dehydrated by sleeping so long and going for over twelve hours without water. I learned to put a glass of water on my nightstand before bedtime so I could sip water during my lengthy sleeping nights without getting out of bed when I awoke so thirsty. The phone rang again after I hung up on a solicitor. I thought to myself, "Why can't these solicitors leave me alone?" I picked up the phone and said, "What do you want?" It was Don's daughter. She was very sweet to me. She asked me how I was doing. I explained to her that I needed to prepare for my afternoon chemotherapy appointment. She then asked if I had the television on, and I replied no, I just got up and I needed to consume a big glass of water because I was dehydrated.

(Apparently my chemotherapy treatment contributed to my dehydration.) Years later I learned that consuming water with electrolytes could help you avoid such dehydration and help you feel more energetic and have less elevation of your blood pressure.

Don's daughter told me a plane had crashed into the World Trade Center in New York City. I was shocked and replied, "You mean a small single engine plane, right?" She said, "No, it was a big American Airlines plane." I was stunned into deep silence. Then she told me to check it out on the television. The damage was extensive. I began to suffer from disbelief that this could happen and turned on the television to view this horrible event which led to the collapse of the World Trade Center where I had spent time when I visited New York City years ago. I drank my glass of water and started to move into action. I thought of the Beatles song "Help." I needed that.

I had planned to work three to four hours that morning. Based on past chemotherapy treatments, I was aware that it could be a week before I felt well enough to accomplish more work. I had certain important tasks to complete. I needed to delegate certain tasks to my assistant who was helping me on these days. The telephone rang at least seven times while I was engaged in my work. Everyone wanted to discuss what was going on in New York. Certain friends who lived in Manhattan called to tell me what was happening and how it affected them. I had to set the phone aside so I could work. I knew about the disaster, and I was facing my own disaster. I concluded I could not control what was going on in New York. I could get control of my own disaster and needed to do so that morning. Then I realized Don was out bicycling and would have no idea what was going on. I tried to call his mobile phone and left a message for him that he would hear when he stopped cycling to take a break. Then I turned to work. Later, Don checked in and asked me questions about the specifics of the 9/11 disaster. Now it was time to listen to the Moody Blues. I listened to "Thinking Is the Best Way to Travel" and "Tuesday Afternoon." The songs comforted me, and I was able to finish my work and then prepare for my afternoon chemotherapy session.

All right, why do I keep naming songs that comfort me? Because music is my life. It allows me to live life fully when I encounter miserable or frightening incidents or attend special events. "Irish" or "Celtic" people have an extensive history of enjoying music, dancing, and laughter. We learn to follow the musical traditions early in our lives. When I was ten years old, I chose "Cecilia" as my confirmation name and then when the bishop appeared at the church service, he gently slapped my face and called me a "soldier of Christ." I believe I still am one more than fifty years later! Now it is time for "My Sweet Lord" by George Harrison of the Beatles.

I had read the book *The Lives of Saints*. It said that St. Cecilia was the patron saint of music. It is time to listen to "Cecilia" by Simon & Garfunkel. I had already studied music theory by the time I was ten years old. At that time, I begged my parents to buy a piano and found one in ads in the newspaper, but it was not possible for them at that time because my father had open heart surgery and there were great worries about his ability to recuperate and return to work. My desire to learn how to play the piano was put on hold. By the time we had one, I was too busy with all my high school activities to devote time to learn how to play the piano. Now it is time to listen to "Your Song" by Elton John.

My brothers helped me learn how to play a guitar. They taught me about the best musical artists and all the great music one could enjoy in the late 1960s including all the wonderful music played at the "Woodstock" concert held in New York State in 1969. Fifty years later, in 2019, I danced for an hour and a half at the local celebration of the anniversary of that event.

In January 2019, I was listening to music on the radio. All of the sudden it was announced that a study had been completed that said rock music kills cancer cells and listening to music during cancer treatments made them more effective! I believe classical music brings joy to soul. That is why Don and I had listened to and enjoyed Beethoven and other artists like Mozart and Tchaikovsky and the opera singer Pavarotti as much as possible. Now it is time to listen to Beethoven's Ninth Symphony, Fourth Movement: "Ode to Joy." Lately, when I listened to that song composed about 250 years ago, I could tell how artists like the Beatles were influenced by classical music when they began their careers.

Ever since January of 2019 I have listened to rock and classical music on my mobile phone as I walked to get my exercise. This helped me enjoy my long walks and extensive exercise to improve my health. When I told someone about my daily walks listening to music, she called it my "Rock Walk."

In 2001, when the afternoon of 9/11 arrived, Don drove me to the nearby oncology office for my chemotherapy treatment. The oncologist examined me. He was one of my favorite doctors because he had worked at the Cleveland Clinic. He was devoted to providing excellent care to me. He was funny and thought the bras I wore were a challenge. Instead of fastening in the back, as he was accustomed to seeing, I wore bras that had special fasteners in the front. He asked me to unfasten my bra. Don always chuckled about his reaction to my different bra. A nurse rushed in to see the oncologist. She said one of the patients was having a problem. He said to her, "Call nine one one, I cannot treat everything myself."

Then, I was seated in the general room where chemotherapy intravenous treatments were administered to patients. I sat in an available reclining chair, and a nurse hooked me up to the IV after she retrieved my "cocktail" of drugs. The nurses were friendly and knowledgeable, so they were special too. When I turned to watch the television that was always played during the lengthy period it took for the IV to be administered, I thought, "Oh no!" It was a constant broadcast about the 9/11 disaster. I thought I had left that behind at home. We watched the news during the hours it took to administer my IV. That was very disturbing and frightening to me. It is too bad I did not know that music, instead of frightening news, could enhance the effectiveness of my chemotherapy treatment. Based on the study results I learned about many years later, I should have insisted on pleasant music instead of the disturbing news about the 9/11 atrocity. Later, when I had my surgery, I would wonder how my last cancer treatment had affected my mind and cancer tumor.

When my chemotherapy session was complete, I was exhausted emotionally and physically. The nurse instructed me to drink clear fluids when I got home. I knew I always needed water after my treatment and drank some before I got up to leave. Then I wanted to retreat to the local Irish pub that was one of our favorite restaurants and a place to enjoy listening to and dancing to live Irish music during our dinner. Before we left, I stopped and asked the nurse if Chardonnay wine was considered a clear fluid. She replied that it was a clear fluid provided I did not consume too much. I always did my best to follow their instructions. Maybe Billy Joel's song "Scenes from an Italian Restaurant" would be fun to hear now.

Don drove us to the Irish pub because I thought a pleasant break would relieve my worries about the victims of 9/11. The owners and servers at the Irish pub were exceptionally friendly and always inquired how my cancer treatments were going. We ordered shepherd's pie, and water, and one glass of wine to drink while we enjoyed songs played by the usual band that played at the Pub, like "Danny Boy" and "Sweet Sixteen" and "Love's Old Sweet Song" and "When Irish Eyes Are Smiling" and "The Town I Loved So Well." The music brought me comfort and joy because I could sing and dance. The single glass of wine was secondary but helped me relax. When we finished our dinner, we went home, and I went to bed because the events of the day had exhausted me.

V. WHAT HAPPENS AFTER SURVIVING CHEMOTHERAPY, HOW DO YOU THRIVE?

When you complete your treatment, it is time to look for a nutritious diet with "whole food" ingredients which are absorbed by your body better than vitamin pills. Of course, you must undergo proper exercise to restore your health and wellness, not to mention completing any necessary surgery to rid yourself of the cancerous tumor. Refer to appendix A and appendix B for suggestions and information about this.

VI. HOW TO ACHIEVE HEALTH, WELLNESS, RECOVERY DURING AND AFTER CHEMOTHERAPY

About two weeks after my chemotherapy treatment, we prepared to fly to Chicago. John Denver's "Fly Away" is pleasant now. I was scheduled for surgery on October 8, 2001, at Northwestern Hospital in Evanston, Illinois, the site of our former home and where my office was when I was operating my legal practice full time. I had to sell my office furniture and have my office files packed and sent to Florida during August because I could not continue to manage the office during my cancer treatment. Before and after my surgery, I continued to serve certain Illinois clients.

When we left Florida, we handed the keys to our condo to the contractor who did a fabulous job of rehabilitating our condo to fix everything damaged by the big water leak from our washer.

Once we arrived in Chicago, we stayed with close friends who were members of the Evanston Bicycle Club, like us. The morning of October 8th, I showed up at the hospital and met with my surgeon, who was the chief of surgery for breast cancer. He was wonderful and took good care of me. He greeted us when we arrived and saw that I was escorted to a room where special scans and tests were administered. After the scans and tests were completed, the surgeon met with a team of doctors who examined the test results to determine my condition. They discussed whether it was better for me to have a mastectomy or if a lumpectomy was appropriate in my case. That day I finally had a victory after a long, hot, unpleasant summer of chemotherapy. Now it was time to listen to "We Are the Champions" by Queen.

I was getting my lumpectomy and not getting my entire right breast destroyed by a mastectomy! I had already decided not to have reconstructive surgery on my right breast. I was concerned about breast implants then because they often interfered with future mammograms to monitor one's cancer status. I had represented certain women involved in the class-action suit when I worked at a Chicago law firm. They had silicone breast implants that appeared to cause additional cancer problems. Saline breast implants were available, but I was not convinced they were a safe alternative. I found a way to get special bras and inserts that made both of my breasts look the same size when I was dressed. Swimsuits offered cups that were sufficient to disguise the fact that my right breast was too small. Now, in 2020, there are alternatives like removing fat and skin from another part of your body and using those items to restore your breast to its former shape. It is time for "Annie's Song" by John Denver.

After the doctors agreed that a lumpectomy was appropriate for me, I was wheeled into surgery. I knew nothing else until I was taken to my inpatient room after surgery was complete. Don and the surgeon briefed me on the results of my surgery as I tried to

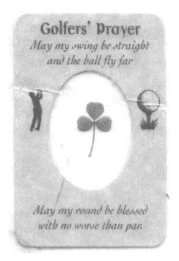

Golfers' Prayer
May my swing be straight
and the ball fly far

May my round be blessed
with no worse than par.

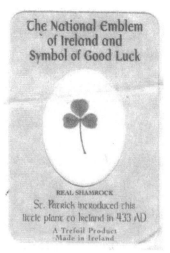

The National Emblem
of Ireland and
Symbol of Good Luck

REAL SHAMROCK
St. Patrick introduced this
little plant to Ireland in 433 AD

A Trefoil Product
Made in Ireland

recover from the anesthesia. I was frightened to hear that they had found cancerous lymph nodes in my right armpit. They removed one third of my lymph nodes under my right arm. Later I would research and learn how the missing lymph nodes would affect my health and how to avoid a serious case of lymphedema that surfaces after removal of lymph nodes.

The surgeon informed me that I would need to have more extensive chemotherapy to ensure there were no cancerous cells left in my body. Later, I would discover that I was facing at least six more months of chemotherapy to supplement the three months of chemotherapy treatment I had completed. I was disappointed by this turn of events because I had thought that when my surgery was completed, I was through with chemotherapy. Plus, I would need six weeks of radiation treatment when I completed the chemotherapy treatment that could have been avoided if I had a radical mastectomy instead of the lumpectomy I had chosen. Now I needed to listen to "It's a Wild World" by Cat Stevens.

A close friend of mine who was a fabulous bicyclist and member of the Evanston Bicycle Club showed up at my hospital room to check up on me and my condition. As she greeted me, I welcomed her, and then suddenly I was vomiting, and it continued for at least twenty minutes. This was how the anesthesia had affected me, I thought. Had the news about cancerous lymph nodes contributed to this? I had never had such lengthy or serious surgery ever in my life before this. No wonder they do not want you to eat or drink for many hours before surgery. If I had consumed anything during my fasting period, this could have happened to me during my surgery! That would have threatened my survival. My friend hung in there with me for a while, and then she bid me farewell and good luck! Time for a special prayer. The Golfer's Prayer from Ireland: "May my swing be straight and the ball fly far. May my round be blessed with no worse than par." Reference to the Shamrock "The National Emblem of Ireland and a Symbol of Good Luck." "St. Patrick introduced this little plant to Ireland in 433 AD." The shamrock plant was made in Ireland. Time to listen to "When Irish Eyes are Smiling" by the Three Irish Tenors.

I was discharged from the hospital by noon the next day. Soon after my discharge, I visited my surgeon. He briefed me again on my future treatment to make sure I understood what was necessary. He examined my wounds and my stitches to make sure I was all right. He made sure I understood how to care for my wounds. It took several more days to recover from my surgical procedure. Once it was determined that I was all right, Don and I packed everything, thanked our good friends for allowing us to stay in their home, and then we flew back to Florida.

I took time off for the rest of October to get properly rested and relaxed before I was to begin my new more aggressive and lengthy chemotherapy treatment. By the first of November, I began my six months of chemotherapy treatments. I still worried whether I could survive such a lengthy treatment, so I prayed to God and hoped for the best. A continuous positive attitude was important to succeed at this type of treatment. I realized that it would be well into the year 2002 before I could even hope to return to a normal life. Time to listen to "Time in a Bottle" by Jim Croce.

By the time my chemotherapy and radiation treatments ended, I would face many years of exams by an oncologist and certain tests and a never-ending need for a digital diagnostic mammogram each year and sometimes a 3D mammogram to ensure any existing breast cancer problem could be identified. These are not the normal breast scans administered to the average woman in order to detect breast cancer early. Now it was time to listen to "Hard-Headed Woman" by Cat Stevens.

When my six months of chemotherapy treatment began, I resolved to exercise daily to try to lose some weight I had gained in the past year and to try to prevent further weight gain. I needed good exercise for both mental and physical relief. After a few chemotherapy sessions, I discovered after talking to my oncologist about my IV treatment that the "cocktail" included what he called "an industrial sized dose of steroids." I remembered that my mother, who was the charge nurse at the VA hospital in Omaha for years, had told me years ago that steroids were not good for me. I was frightened when I was told it was an "industrial-sized dose." Because my oncologist knew about my fears and anxiety concerning chemotherapy and because my more "aggressive" treatment would last at least twice as long as the initial treatment before surgery, I told him I was very worried and wanted to have steroids removed from my "IV cocktail."

My oncologist contacted other oncologists throughout the country to see if cancer patients like me had been able to survive well without the "industrial-sized dose" of steroids. It took some time. Within a couple weeks he had received certain information, and he informed me that he thought my treatment could be successful without the steroid dose. So, my IV cocktail was altered, and I was ready to resume my chemotherapy treatment. Now it is time for "I Am a Rock" by Simon and Garfunkel.

When I went to my next chemotherapy treatment, the nurse said my veins were collapsing from all the IV treatments. She had to insert the IV needle between my toes on my left foot. Then she recommended a special surgeon to consult about having a port placed in my chest so the IV treatment could be properly administered for the remainder of my treatment. I met with the surgeon and he arranged for me to have surgery at the hospital. I went as an out-patient for surgery. Waiting for surgery, experiencing it, and recovering took almost all day. When I finished, I was starved, because I fasted a long time before the surgery. When I was released from the hospital, we drove to the nearby McDonald's, and I ate a quarter pounder with cheese. I do not remember ever having another one because it is pretty fattening. Plus, I found out consuming food from McDonald's did not help you to avoid cancer.

Now, I was ready for my next treatment. The next concern about my chemotherapy treatment was that I experienced constant vomiting in the mornings after I received treatment. I was worried about how sick the treatment made me feel and called the nurses at the hematology clinic. They said, "You cannot skip a treatment because you feel sick. You need to come whenever you are scheduled." I said, "Okay, how do I survive this treatment?" They told me: "Follow our diet." It was called the "BRAT" diet. B stood for banana. The R stood for rice. The A stood for Applesauce. The T stood for toast. This would give me potassium and fiber without consuming large portions of food and would keep my stomach calm, which would relieve me from such awful side effects. I followed the BRAT diet, and it worked for me.

When I finally finished chemotherapy treatment, the oncologist prescribed a popular medicine for cancer patients: Tamoxifen. He said I needed it to survive. I took the medicine for several weeks. I vomited after each meal and felt miserable and wondered how I could ensure I was getting proper nutrition. I told him, "No more, I cannot take it; I cannot survive this way." The oncologist said: "Some cancer patients survived without taking Tamoxifen." So, I resolved to stop taking it and was ready to face up to the consequences. I had my port removed by the surgeon then because my chemotherapy treatment had ended.

Now it was time to start six weeks of radiation treatment, which was performed every weekday. I went to the radiologist, and she measured my chest, neck, and shoulders. Then they tried to position the radiation machine. There was a pause, and little blue tattoos were placed on my chest to help each technician line up the radiation properly for me. Extra care was taken around my neck so my thyroid gland would not be affected. At that point I had been taking medicine for hypothyroidism for about eighteen years. I had a rare form called "Hashimoto's thyroiditis" that meant extra care was needed. The blue tattoos looked like little blue freckles, and they are still apparent on my chest, twenty years later. I was told to stay out of the sun and get plenty of rest because I was likely to experience significant fatigue because of the radiation treatment. I paid attention to this advice and survived the radiation with flying colors.

Within two weeks after I completed my treatment, I realized it was almost a year since I had detected the large tumor on my right breast, and unlike my father, I had weathered and avoided severe side effects of the treatment, so far. I had survived about nine months of chemotherapy and one and a half months of radiation, plus three different surgeries. Now I wonder if "survival" is possible under these circumstances when you reach an age over sixty-five because anesthesia and surgery is very difficult for aged persons to survive.

Don and I flew to Ireland for specially arranged tour, and two other cancer "survivors" accompanied us on the tour. The flight was uneventful, but I experienced significant fatigue after we arrived at the hotel. Some of that was due to "jet lag" even though I slept on the plane and followed certain dietary rules to avoid severe jet lag. I rested as much as possible, and some of the time I suggested to others that they take the bus tour of the nearby area without me on certain days so that I could rest. I participated in the special events at the hotel much of the time and enjoyed the music and some dancing for exercise. I made sure I had plenty of rest before we were scheduled to attend a luncheon at a nearby Irish castle. The food was fabulous. There was live music. Of course, that is how the Irish live, love, and laugh. It was a great break from my worries about my fatigue following the radiation. Time to listen to "Will You Go Lassie Go?" by the Irish Tenors.

One day we took time off the tour and traveled to Patrickswell in County Limerick in western Ireland to visit my Irish cousins who I had gotten to know well between 1985 and 1996 and not been able to visit them since 1996. My cousin, who owned and managed a bed and breakfast (B&B) inn treated us to Irish soda bread, which she had taught me how to make. We enjoyed tea while we snacked. Then other cousins made a toast to me and encouraged me to recover from my cancer treatment. When they toasted me, they said: "Slainte," and I asked them what that meant. They said it was Gaelic for "Cheers." I would use that word to make a toast to friends for many years to come.

By 2018 I found out a couple cousins died of Alzheimer's, and I was sad and wondered if my mother or I would suffer from that eventually. See the appendix of this book for publications concerning dietary suggestions to avoid Alzheimer's. In 2018 the cousin who owned the B&B died too. When I found that out, I purchased a special Irish soda bread loaf pan that I use to make the Irish soda bread like she made, and I make it often in her memory. Time to listen to "Amazing Grace" and "Nearer My God to Thee" by the Irish Tenors.

We returned to the hotel where we were staying with other tour participants. We enjoyed the rest of the tour immensely and I was less fatigued. One place where we stopped to shop had special handmade and hand-painted statues that I purchased. Plus, I found a special CD of Irish music. I still listen to it regularly eighteen years later. It is called "Celtic Airs," and the cover says it is "A unique collection of traditional Irish melodies, rich in texture and color like the Irish landscape itself." That is why I knew I would enjoy it when I returned home. Time to listen to the melody "Women of Ireland." Next, we prepared to fly home.

VII. OVERCOMING THE EFFECTS OF CHEMOTHERAPY ON THE MIND AND BODY

After my cancer treatment in 2001 and 2002, I had significant weight gain, and it was hard to understand how it happened. I kept a detailed journal to record my diet, exercise, weight, and measurement of certain parts of my body. I worked so hard to lose weight and could not do it! I tried many different approaches and failed. I felt fat and hated it. I had tried to stay trim my entire life. I wondered if it was related to the lymphedema I tried so hard to avoid. Finally, after so much effort, I decided to resort to liposuction, for me a last resort because it required surgery and treatment by a plastic surgeon! I felt better after the treatment. Many years later, when I attended my forty-fifth high school reunion, I got a Swedish massage, a facial, my hair trimmed and styled, and manicured my nails and got dressed up for the event. Don remarked to one of my classmates that I appeared to be the "best dressed" one at the reunion. Almost everyone came in casual dress. After we took pictures of all the classmates in attendance, one of my male classmates said to Don that "Marianne always was a dandy!" It is time for "You Are So Beautiful" by Joe Cocker.

Chemotherapy had a serious effect on how my brain worked. I had a "foggy" brain and had difficulty with my memory and concentration. Two years after the treatment had ended, I still had so much difficulty that I could not look forward to the full-time practice of law. When you begin a new practice, you need to plan full time, and that often means a challenging investment of time and effort requiring solid brain activity. When I discussed my frustration with a friend, she suggested I try to sell real estate instead of practicing law until my recovery was more complete. She was in the real estate business and owned a school to assist people to prepare for and pass the real estate exam to get a realtor's license in Florida. I considered her suggestion carefully and concluded I could be a part-time realtor without working excessive hours or having extraordinary demands that required a fully operational brain for me. I also thought that entering the real estate business would help me get to know Florida better.

I attended her school and learned the important things needed to pass the realtor's examination. I passed on the first try, and before I knew it, she recommended that a realtor friend of hers hire me, so I was able to get a position without tons of work and started my position soon after I had passed the exam. I learned a lot about the purchase and sale contracts and rental contracts. Certain agents working at the same firm helped me master the sales techniques. Others learned about my ability to master the requirements and fulfill client expectations for leasing out their home or condominium when they migrated to the north for a good portion of the year. They referred clients to me, and I honored their request not to engage in sale of their clients' real properties and worked only on leases.

A very experienced realtor at the firm where I worked heard me discussing issues with sales and leases and gave me some good advice and invited me to view certain new communities with her to learn enough to engage in sales. She assisted me with a new client I had taken on to sell their house for them and gave me excellent guidance. She took me "under her wing," and when she found out I was a cancer survivor, she invited me to participate with her in raising money for the "Sunshine Kids," which was dedicated to helping children who had cancer. When we joined forces, we were able to raise a good amount for that cause.

Working as a real estate agent helped me to gain more confidence in how my brain operated, and the concentration required for the work improved my ability to concentrate and achieve my goals and objectives. After working for a couple of years, I found an excellent preparation course for the Florida bar examination. I attended all the lectures and took sample exams and received CDs that contained all the lectures so I could listen to the lectures several times and review all the most important materials to prepare for the exam. I came to understand that repetition was a key strategy to learn how to sit for and pass the exam. I prayed to God, and She made sure I was able to pass the exam.

I finally passed the exam in October 2006 and was hired by an excellent attorney by the beginning of January 2007. This was a fabulous achievement, and I finally was able to return to the full-time practice of law. I had maintained my Illinois practice on a part-time basis, but now I had mastered the laws I needed to know to return to a full-time position. My brain, body, and life had finally been renewed about five years after my cancer treatment had begun!

A few years later I decided to establish my own legal practice. Now is the time to listen to "My Way" by Frank Sinatra. It was challenging to go back to my own practice because I needed certain office space and assistance and needed to work on marketing. I joined an attorneys' networking group and the American Business-woman Association (known as ABWA) to help me achieve my goals. Within several years, after I successfully established my own practice, I had more critical health issues that affected my work. Even with special rehabilitation advice I still had great difficulty.

I had to resolve health issues like diabetes so that eventually I learned the wrong dose of one medicine which was too high (levothyroxine for hypothyroidism) probably caused this problem; and I suffered from awful side effects from prescription medicines I had been taking for years, weight problems I had to resolve, and certain kind of scary symptoms that appeared to be related to Parkinson's. I had so many health issues to deal with, after a few years I finished all my work and closed and stored certain client files. Then I decided I was forced to retire from the Illinois and Florida attorneys' (not drinking) bar associations. This made me miserable to believe I may not recover or ever be able to work again. I did lots of research and looked for solutions to all these problems. I kept my brain as active as possible and focused on getting rest and relaxation so that I could try to recover.

It took me over three years to recover and prepare myself to begin working again as a Florida bar attorney. I did it, and within a year or so, I made major progress in establishing a new legal practice. What a challenge! What a relief! IT IS DEFINITELY TIME TO LISTEN TO "THE IMPOSSIBLE DREAM" as sung by one of the three Irish Tenors (Ronan Tynan) I listen to very often to help me achieve calmness and happiness.

The most important news to disclose now follows: In the last twenty years I had identified ways to overcome at least seven different chronic illnesses that had affected my legal career. Now I was finally able to practice again at a level I had not fully achieved for the last eighteen years! I had conducted careful research about how to resolve the "root causes" of my health problems and ways to identify medical providers who could truly help me. I had resolved many problems by indicating to my medical providers that my focus was on how to treat the root cause of problems and not take endless medicines that only treated the "effects" of my health problems because the prescription medicines in almost every instance were substantially contributing to my inability to fully recover. Again, when my husband witnessed all my efforts and the conclusions I had reached, he continued to call me "Dr. C" even though I do not possess a medical doctor's license. Once again, I am an "AAD" ("Almost A Doctor"). I am a juris doctor (JD), not an MD. Some people might consider me a "witch doctor."

VIII. LEARNING HOW TO LIVE MY LIFE MORE FULLY DURING AND AFTER CANCER TREATMENT

The first week of January 2019 had momentous events for me. The ear, nose, and throat doctor attended to my new hearing aide. After fifty-five years, I could hear things on the right side of my body. I saw an oncologist who promised me certain important cancer tests to "rid me of the fear of cancer," and they were supposed to happen as soon as possible. In January, the oncologist's staff asserted I did not qualify for a mammogram under my insurance so soon after my screening mammogram in November 2018. I told them politely they were not well informed and that because I had obtained a better, new health plan that had become effective at the beginning of January 2019, I knew I qualified for the tests that they were not acting promptly to schedule. This was causing a lot of anxiety as I continued to worry from mid-January through February. Time to listen to Billy Joel sing "Only the Good Die Young."

By the end of February (about six weeks later) I had not had the most important cancer tests I needed since my cancer diagnosis almost eighteen years earlier! I contacted the provider who was supposed to help schedule the test and spoke to someone who was in charge. When I told her that I was a frequent performer of yoga, she called me a pretzel! She was nice and had a good sense of humor.

The oncologist and his staff from the locally based Cancer Institute had failed to respond after *four weeks* to a provider's request to clarify a doctor's order concerning my cancer tests, especially an ultrasound on my pancreas. The need for the ultrasound of my pancreas worried me because I had overcome diabetes several years earlier and my uncle had died of pancreatic cancer. I always worried about my potential for illnesses like my relatives had because I figured my genetic make-up might mean I could have similar health issues. These days, getting genetic testing can help your oncologist identify possible health problems arising because of damage to your DNA. Sharing such genetic test results with family members can also help them pursue proper treatment. Time to listen to "I Can't Keep It In" by Cat Stevens.

When I investigated this myself near the end of February, I discovered this terrible neglect of my healthcare and needs, and my healing lymphedema went WILD! I was furious that I had been put in this awful situation. I voiced my displeasure vociferously with the oncologist's staff. THE ONCOLOGIST HAD THE NERVE TO TELL MY PSYCHOLOGIST I WAS OUT OF CONTROL. Who wouldn't be if their care had been so terribly neglected and they were facing possible serious cancer concerns that were valid based on the oncologist's advice? Billy Joel's "Just the Way You Are" is meaningful now.

A close friend had died in early 2018 after she had not pursued proper tests and treatment concerning possible cancer disease early enough. Would that happen to me as well? The truth is that the oncologist and his staff at the local Cancer Institute were out of control! I have continuously wondered how a major contributor to the Cancer Institute would feel about that. Read on for more detail. It was time to listen to the Three Irish Tenors sing "Only Our Rivers Run Free" to help me calm down. My Irish music was always a way to calm myself, in addition to visiting my psychologist and making an entry in my personal journal that I had kept for the last twenty years to help relieve frustration and health concerns.

I soon recalled the following statement I had seen a long time ago about medical treatment. "Doctors pour drugs, of which they know little, to cure diseases, of which they know less, into human beings, of which they know nothing." That statement has stuck with me for over thirty years!

I felt abused by this oncologist and his staff, who knew NOTH-ING about me and never even tried to learn about who I was and what kind of cancer fears I was enduring. I spent considerable time with my psychologist to overcome my fear and deep anxiety they caused. I felt like I was being punished for some reason by the medical staff. Was this related to the Health Department complaint I filed against another doctor who failed to properly administer a doctor's order for a brain MRI? His staff tried to charge me for a test that was never properly administered and which he had promised me at the time he ended the MRI before completion that I would not be charged. I tried to resolve the issue informally, and they acted in an unreasonable fashion, in my opinion, because they threatened me with collection action for a test that was never completed properly. They left me with no choice but to report the doctor to the Department of Health not long before his license was up for renewal. *Plus, in 2016 he had reported normal results from that MRI "test" that was never completed to my neurologist who was treating me for Parkinson's symptoms at that time. Was it not possible to get good treatment in Delray Beach, Florida, now? Maybe not.*

After I expressed my extreme displeasure with the oncologist's treatment of me by his staff, they finally made my appointments for a mammogram and the ultrasound of my pancreas. The oncologist had said after my CT scan in early January that he had concerns about cancer of my pancreas. This caused great anxiety while I waited many weeks for the scheduling of the proper testing because my uncle, who was my godfather, had died of pancreatic cancer! A rule of thumb for me based on the people I knew who were deceased due to cancer follows: GET EXAMINED AND GET

PROPER TESTING AS SOON AS POSSIBLE SO THERE CAN BE REMEDIES PURSUED AS EARLY AS POSSIBLE TO AVOID DEATH! I told a friend how worried I was about too big of a delay in getting my testing completed because a dear friend had died the year before my testing after she had failed to pursue proper testing and care early enough to avoid death.

When the oncologist's staff scheduled the appointments in a big hurry because of my great anxiety about the delay in testing, they FAILED TO OBTAIN AUTHORIZATION FOR THE TESTS FROM MY HEALTH INSURANCE COMPANY. An authorization was not a difficult or a time-consuming task for proper medical professionals, but they clearly did not care about me and maybe they were not properly informed about my insurance plan and coverage. They had not listened to my explanations about my coverage and had not checked with my primary insurance carrier about the so-called "coverage issues." Because I did not trust them, I checked with my insurance company as soon as possible after I was notified about the "appointment" for the cancer testing. The insurance company informed me the tests had NOT been authorized. I would have paid many hundreds of dollars for these tests if I showed up. I CANCELLED THESE BOGUS APPOINT-MENTS when I found out that they would not be properly covered by my health insurance plan.

Because my cancer care was neglected and my anxiety and lymphedema became as bad as it gets, I "fired" the Florida doctor from the Cancer Institute and went to a different Florida doctor who had cared for me for years before. He and his wonderful staff helped me and got my tests scheduled and authorized within two business days (instead of the many weeks I had already experienced)! I had already waited at least sixteen weeks since my "screening mammo-gram" that was done in November of 2018 because of cancer questions arising due to the sudden arrival of my severe lymphedema which had caused problems that necessitated a couple visits to a hospital emergency room in the autumn of 2018 and several treatments at a lymphatics clinic.

I was on a new health plan in 2019, and I had made sure the health plan would cover the digital diagnostic mammogram, a 3D mammogram, an ultrasound of my pancreas before I agreed to use it. So, now I just paid my normal insurance copayment. Thank the Lord that my doctor and his staff cared for me properly and the provider who administered the tests conducted thorough testing as well.

The Florida oncologist pronounced me cancer free in early March, but I never believed him or trusted him based on what I described above. The women's clinic where I was tested said I should see a dermatologist about the bumps on my skin (I thought I might have skin cancer). The clinic also sent me a letter saying if I had any doubts about breast cancer to have a breast MRI. My oncologist never suggested I obtain those tests. Do you see why I do not trust him or his staff? It took time and commitment by me to obtain all the correct tests during 2019. During the time I waited and worried about whether I would be a "survivor" if I did not resolve all my doubts. Billy Joel's "She's Got A Way" means something to me now.

During January 2019, Don made an offer on a condo in the same building we had lived in for almost three years. We thought by moving to a larger apartment I would be able to handle more tasks, and ensure I had greater privacy from members of the community board of directors who visited Don at home. I believed I needed a more spacious apartment for privacy so that I could heal my lymphedema better. I had prayed to God for healing, and he was answering my prayers! I worked full time for Don for three weeks to get him a mortgage loan and close on the new apartment he purchased. We were ready to close on the purchase before the end of February. Then, I paid a mover hundreds of dollars to pack and move our household goods and furniture to the new, larger apartment because I was physically unable to accomplish packing and moving household items up to the second floor of the building we had lived in for three years.

My right arm had become swollen and painful due to lymphedema and the fear and anxiety I faced as described above. I could not undertake a move without assistance of this mover. It would be many weeks before I could unpack all the boxes of household goods. I was sick the day the movers came. They did not accomplish as much as I had hoped. I could not supervise the move well because I spent so much time in bed resting. Later during early April, I would have to complete the move of certain items with the help of a neighbor who understood what I was going through. He and his wife were thankful for certain help I had given them and gave me a gift of love. Now it is time to listen to "Moving Out" by Billy Joel.

By the way, because of my experience in 2001, when I discovered I had breast cancer thirty days after a complex move from Illinois, I always seem to believe that when I undertake a move of my residence or office that I might be getting cancer again. A mental trauma I will always have difficulty overcoming. Now, after getting psychological therapy, I believe I have found some way to achieve lasting psychological recovery. *2019 was a disastrous year because I undertook two residence moves and three quick and difficult office moves! No one understands the trauma I experienced for most of 2018 through 2020 because of blood pressure, stroke, and cancer scares and the residence and office moves I accomplished because I HAD NO CHOICE!*

After we had moved most of our belongings to the new apartment in late February, I petitioned the Florida bar to reinstate my bar license. I was forced to give up my bar license and retire from the Florida bar in 2017 because I had been disabled since 2015 and I believed I would never be able to return to the practice of law given my severe health problems at that time. I was also concerned from 2015–2018 whether I would survive the terrible chronic illnesses I had.

In early March 2019, I had completed all the necessary continuing legal education to obtain my Florida bar license again when I had spent full-time hours for weeks assisting my husband with his legal and financial needs. After I obtained my license, I told a friend about all the work I had done even at 3:00 and 4:00 a.m. to accomplish my goals, and she called me the "ENERGIZER BUNNY." Now it is time to listen to "The Night Is Still Young" by Billy Joel.

In 2015 a neurologist thought I had Parkinson's symptoms and referred me to a specialist that I saw in 2016, and he examined me and arranged for special brain scans to see how serious my illness might be. By late 2016 I had sufficiently changed my lifestyle and diet to rid myself of my diabetes diagnosis, and six years after my diagnosis, I was no longer insulin dependent. I had lost fifty pounds since 2010 and returned to my high school weight. My fasting glucose level was so low I would have been in the emergency room if I took any insulin.

Then in 2017, I had three serious falls. I had osteoporosis because of my early menopause during chemotherapy treatment. When I stood up after a test at the mammogram clinic, I twisted my ankle, lost my balance, and broke my ankle and leg. The ankle surgeon congratulated me when he determined I did not need surgery and could heal if I wore a special cast for a couple months. After my serious falls, a nurse advised me that I should get special physical therapy to ensure my neck and shoulders were strong enough to prevent me from breaking my neck. I did it. It is time for "The Prayer of Protection" recited at Unity of Delray Beach.

Nobody but Don understood the continuing health problems I had experienced since 2014 and earlier and how much my life was impacted during the last five years or so by these health conditions. I worked hard to read books and educate myself and try to find a way to recover. I never openly complained about my health concerns, so most people did not understand what I was going through.

I took the necessary continuing legal education credits in late February and early March in 2019. I paid my dues. By March 12, 2019, I received my certificate of good standing, demonstrating that I had completed all the requirements to reinstate my Florida bar license. This was not a simple task. I had many conversations with Florida bar membership staff to resolve questions about my status. At one point when I had completed all the necessary credits and had not gotten my license, I asked a staff member who my lawyer should contact so I could be awarded my license. (I did not have a lawyer!) The next day, I had my license. Do you see how being assertive and mildly aggressive in certain circumstances can benefit you, legally? Billy Joel's song "Big Shot" is meaningful now.

On March 15th I was warned that certain individuals in my community wanted to "POP me!" I instantly reacted by saying if someone killed me, my husband would know to bring a wrongful death action. Of course, if such threats were carried out, those persons would have committed premeditated murder! When I found out about those threats, Don was visiting people in Boca Raton. I called him and told him what I had learned and that he needed to come to our "home" and take me elsewhere because of my fear that I could be killed. When he came home, I threw my clothes, shoes, and jewelry in a suitcase in a big hurry because I did not know when I would return "home."

We went to Unity of Delray Beach and I prayed for peace and harmony. It is time to sing "Let there be peace and let it begin with me…" Don called his sister who made a reservation for us at the lodge in her secure gated community. We did not know where else I would feel safe and secure at this point. Early on March 16th, Don came to visit me after spending the previous evening and that morning caring for my cat Pearl for me. We talked about my life experiences for two hours after his arrival early in the morning and certain past events that had led to happiness for me. When I got up to go for a walk and retreat to the restaurant for breakfast, I almost fell over. I hobbled back to the bed and told Don my heart was racing, and if I got up, I thought I might fall and break my neck. This was less than twenty-four hours after I found out that certain people had threatened to "POP" me! Time to listen to the song "Peace Train" by Cat Stevens.

I told Don that I thought I might be having a stroke. I could feel my heart racing! The community had paramedics who came and took my blood sugar and gave me an EKG. They said my blood sugar was normal and that I had the "heart of a fifteen-year-old."

But I felt so awful. They said I should go to the emergency room for certain tests that they could not administer.

Because of my fear, I took an aspirin, hoping if I had a stroke, I would not have severe affects like the paralysis my grandmother experienced because of her first stroke when I was about five years old and suffered from for many years before her ultimate death because of a sudden stroke. About an hour later, the ambulance arrived and took me to the hospital emergency room. My stroke fear was not imagined. I had two grandparents who had died suddenly from strokes. Plus, what if my racing heart was indicative of an approaching heart attack? Another grandfather and my special uncle had died suddenly from heart attacks. What was I going to do? Could I survive?

When we got to the emergency room, the nurse who administered "care" said improper things about me, and I overheard her comments and let her know she was mistaken. While I was resting in the emergency room, Don and I were talking. My niece called me to check in. When I told her that people wanted to POP me, she paused for half a minute, and then she said, "Do you mean they wanted to kill you?" She grew up in Nebraska, as I did, and her father was a deputy sheriff. She had the same reaction I did. Don had been trying to say that "pop" means they did not want to do any more than punch me in the nose so he could minimize these so-called threats. I handed him my cell phone so he could get the truth from my niece.

I endured my "care" at the emergency room for about six or more hours. A doctor stopped and asked me certain questions that did not make much sense to me. We quickly discovered she had stopped at the wrong emergency room bed. Soon after I arrived at the emergency room, I had told the nurse that I had not eaten since 4:00 p.m. the previous day and I wondered if that was contributing to the dizziness I was experiencing. No medical professionals were nearby when I needed to go to the ladies' room, so help was not available for me to walk down the hallway, and I was worried I could fall and be seriously injured because of my dizziness, so I grasped the bars on the wall in the hallway when I was forced to go the ladies' room so that I would not fall because of my dizziness. About six hours went by before I was admitted to the hospital for a stay in which they planned to observe me and make sure I did not have a stroke or require surgery to prevent my possible death. My blood pressure was excessively high and had been for at least seven and a half hours that day.

I did not get food until I was finally moved to an inpatient bed in the hospital. At that point it had been about twenty-two hours since I had last eaten (the day before) when I spoke to a friend on the phone and a nurse in the room who was assisting the patient that I was sharing the room with overheard me say to my friend that I had not eaten for twenty-two hours. Suddenly, the nurse appeared with a plate of food for me! The doctors had wondered why I was dizzy before I was finally fed!

I did not sleep all night. The patient I shared a room with had suffered from a stroke and was screaming in pain and terror all night. By 3:00 a.m. I called the charge nurse in the hospital and complained that this woman needed proper treatment and help, now! The next thing I knew, a nurse came running down the hallway to my roommate's bed. Her screams and apparently her pain seemed to be controlled better, and then she slept. I did not. I needed to hear "Hotel California" by the Eagles now. A special author wrote in a book called *Take Control of Your Life*: "If you think you are in hell, keep moving..." I could not. I believe that you must keep moving so the devil does not catch up to you and harm you!

Soon after 3:00 a.m., a phlebotomist came to draw my blood for various tests. I had to stop her from puncturing my right arm with a needle. I was suffering severe lymphedema from my cancer treatment eighteen years earlier. I calmly and quietly explained to her that I had told every nurse I had seen that day that my right arm was unavailable for needle sticks or blood pressure because of my lymphedema. I quietly told her that I did not want her to regret sticking a needle in my arm and harming the arm that I had protected for eighteen years. She was upset that no nurse had pre-

71

viously marked my arm to prevent harm to me. It was fortunate that I was awake and aware enough to prevent harm to my right arm! The phlebotomist made sure my arm was not further harmed by placing a special bracelet on it to prevent needle sticks and blood pressure tests. Then she drew my blood in my left arm and bid me farewell. She was one of the few nurses in that hospital who had cared for me!

Around eight in the morning, I complained to the charge nurse about my inadequate care over the past twenty-four hours. I complained that my mother had been a nurse for over forty years and that she had served as a charge nurse at the veterans' hospital as well. I knew what nurses should do. It had been twenty-four hours, and no nurse had provided me with items to make sure I was properly bathed. I worried about bacteria making my lymphedema worse. Within a few minutes, the charge nurse made sure I had the materials to clean myself up! It was clear that he really cared about me!

It was clear to me that many of the nurses on that floor had been improperly trained, had too much work, or just did not care for me. Not one of them responded to my pressing a button for their assistance, so I had to make it in and out of the bathroom by myself even though they knew I was at risk for falling. Then a nurse complained that I could not go there by myself and they needed to administer a urine test. I suggested to the nurse that she bring me whatever was necessary for me to capture my urine when I went to the bathroom without her assistance so they could perform the necessary urine test. I asked why no nurse had responded to requests for assistance, including providing information promised to me about side effects of medications I was being given. I did not get a proper response from her.

I felt like I was being punished for my reasonable comments and complaints to the charge nurse. Almost one year later, at another hospital, I realized most hospital patients did not understand what the charge nurse was and how much you could do when you needed to get proper care by contacting the charge nurse. My mother had been one. So, I was aware and educated other patients so they could get proper care.

Early in the morning I was told that I needed an intravenous ("IV") treatment, and they brought the equipment and set it next to my right arm that was visibly affected by lymphedema and the IV could not be inserted in my right arm. The nurses failed to attempt to hook up the "IV" for many hours, not until well after noon that day. Then they said I could not be discharged that day because I had not had the intravenous treatment. They were trying to punish me and make me stay another full day with no sleep. NO WAY!

It was Sunday, March 17th, St. Patrick's Day. After 8:00 a.m. no one came to bring me breakfast. I called Don and told him to stop and get me breakfast at one of our favorite restaurants. I had been there about twenty-four hours and had lost four pounds! At some point I missed not being able to go to Unity of Delray Beach for church. I cried out in bed, "GOD, HELP ME, HELP ME." Don told me the nurses wanted to call security. I responded, "WHY, BECAUSE I BELIEVE IN GOD?" I have learned at Unity to "Let Go and Let God..." Friends came to visit. We listened to Amazon music on my cell phone and sang songs. Then, the family of my roommate who I had protected by getting her proper care in the wee hours of the morning complained about the music and singing of my visitors and me. Then we sung "My Way" by Frank Sinatra and stopped the music and singing.

Then I called my insurance company and complained about my lack of proper treatment and if I needed more hospital care, I wanted approval to be transferred to a different nearby hospital. Because I had been so insistent on protecting myself that day, the doctor finally agreed to discharge me from the hospital late in the afternoon.

PRAISE THE LORD FOR ANSWERING MY PRAYERS. THEY COULD NOT ARRANGE FOR MY DEATH NOW! Later I would tell Don that I would NOT go to any Florida hospital again. If I needed care, I would take a non-stop flight to Chicago instead!

He became very worried about me after the comment I made that I would not go to a Florida hospital again because they would KILL ME! Later we discussed if I truly needed emergency hospital care, that arrangements should be made to ensure I would only end up at the Cleveland Clinic of Florida because I trusted the care they administered. This would take time to accomplish. Time to listen to "She's Always A Woman" by Billy Joel.

Soon after I was discharged from the hospital on St. Patrick's Day, my brother, who found out about my experiences, drove for two days from Illinois to our home in southeastern Florida to take care of me. He and Don drove me everywhere because the large bandaging on my lymphedema arm prevented me from driving safely. After a lymphatics clinic appointment, my brother and I went to the Dune Deck in Lantana for a pleasant low-calorie lunch. Then we walked down the stairs from the restaurant to the beach where I had to limit my exposure to the sun, but my brother was able to enjoy the ocean waves and water. As we climbed up the stairs from the beach near the parking lot, a woman asked me why I had my huge compression bandage on my right arm. I told her that people in my community had caused me trauma and she said I could not let that happen. I replied that I was working on that! Time to sing along to the Pina Colada Song entitled "Escape" by Rupert Holmes.

Then, I asked her why she was at the beach alone that day. She said she was celebrating her birthday by herself. She told me her father had once been the king of Spain and her mother was Sophia Loren. She had been adopted early in her life and did not know who her parents were until after she reached age fifty. I felt bad for her when she described recent experiences. She was so nice; she deserved to celebrate her birthday with others, and maybe she was a bit lonely that day. It is time to play and sing along to "Happy Birthday, Baby..." by the Tune Weavers.

Then I took her to the bar that was a few steps away and bought her a shot of tequila. I taught her to say "Slainte" when we toasted to her birthday because I had decided to drink some Irish cream. I enjoyed Irish cream, an Irish cordial that was more cream than liquor. The ingredients included a small amount of Irish whiskey and white wine. Most of it was the taste of cream. Now it was time to listen to "Happy Birthday, Baby," a one-hit wonder from the 1950s. Then, my brother drove me home. Time to listen to "Uptown Girl" by Billy Joel. I seem to remember that song was about Christy Brinkley, the daughter of a TV news reporter named David Brinkley.

By March 19th, I contacted two attorneys who told me that the community's board of directors should have called the police or Palm Beach sheriff's office to investigate who had threatened to POP me and do something to protect me. It never happened, and I believe so because it was possibly a board member who wanted to POP me! I did not make a fuss because Don was a board member, and I would not allow him to be impacted if I made a fuss.

I was a hostage in my own apartment. I would not go to the gym, the clubhouse activities, the pool, or for a nature walk. Because of my inability to exercise and my terrible fear of being attacked, I could not exercise there to try to control my horrible blood pressure that had never been this worrisome before my hospitalization in March 2019. Don's cousins saved me. They allowed me to stay in their apartment while they were not residing there. They were snowbirds and would not return for some time. I could sleep, exercise, and eat at their apartment for weeks to come. Then, Don insisted I come home to help him get his apartment listed for sale. Time to listen to "Moving Out" by Billy Joel.

At the end of March, Don and I were guests of his sister at a certain gated community. We went to swim, and then we went to the lounge where they were serving appetizers and fruit-filled cocktails. We each had only one drink. It was a party for the golfers. We learned about certain condo apartments for sale, and I contacted our real estate agent. On April 1st, which was April Fool's Day, we looked at several condos. On April 2nd, I signed a contract to purchase a condo at 6:00 a.m. Believe me, I did not think I was fool at that time. More than a year later, I have begun to think a little differently based on significantly poor treatment by certain males in the community who found out I was a feminist.

The sellers signed the contract the same day, and I qualified for the sixty-two-and-under promotion for free golf dues for a year because I would not turn sixty-three until the next day! This saved us money for our first year while I continued to be rehabilitated for my serious lymphedema problem with my right arm. I had realized that I needed to become left-handed to get through this problem. It is tough to become a "south paw" when you have been right-handed for at least sixty-two years! Time to listen to "Bridge Over Troubled Water" by Simon & Garfunkel.

Yet Another Serious Traumatic Incident to Overcome

On May 2,, 2019, disaster struck. Less than thirty days after I had signed the lease for my new office space, I arrived at my office, turned on the lights, my computer, the printer. Then I went to the lounge to get my cup of green tea, which assists with digestive issues and has important antioxidants. When I returned to my office, my computer, my brand-new printer, and desk were full of water due to water leaking from the roof into the building and through my ceiling. I reported this to the landlord's representative, unplugged and moved my equipment under the desk thinking it would be safe. There was no way to complete important work now or even for two full months, as it turned out. Sometimes I wonder whether the contractor recommendation for the landlord to run a dehumidifier in my office weeks later contributed to harm to my computer. Not only that, when I spent limited time in the office after "repairs" were "made," I went home allergic and congested. Perhaps that meant mold and mildew were rampant in my office and causing an allergic reaction!

I had to transact business in my car on my Android phone for the rest of the day, which was stressful. I had planned to talk to the insurance agent that day about contents insurance for my office when I got homeowners' insurance for my new condo purchase. Now it was out of the question because of the water intrusion event that morning. Now I would face huge delays in accomplishing work, getting new equipment and software so I could transact my business and take care of my personal bill payments. This was a major disaster. I now believe the landlord should have disclosed roof problems to me when I signed the lease and did not do so. I may pursue an action against the owner of the building, not the same as the landlord, because I believe the owner was liable for gross negligence by not seeing that the roof had been properly maintained for the past twenty years.

The day after the water intrusion event, on May 3rd, I experienced extremely high blood pressure. I got a blood pressure monitor after my hospitalization in mid-March for nearly having a stroke so that I could monitor my blood pressure daily. I had not gotten a new prescription for blood pressure medication, which had been prescribed when I was discharged from the hospital, because of the bad side effects, which led to ankle and leg swelling, which seemed to cause pain when I went on a walk for my important exercise routine. I did not think I needed the meds anymore until the water intrusion event on May 2nd. I begged Don to give me some of his medications on May 3rd because I feared I would have a stroke. My doctor prescribed good medications by the end of the weekend, and I survived. Do you now see why my husband Don calls me "Dr. C" frequently? I reminded him I do not have a license as a medical doctor, only a juris doctor. A friend said I am an "AAD." I asked, "What is that?" She said: "You are Almost A Doctor." Now it is time to listen to "My Life" by Billy Joel.

In late August 2019, when we prepared for Hurricane Dorian. I became concerned about how I would be able to accomplish important work I had planned and how I could ensure I had sufficient equipment to accomplish various tasks. We grocery shopped based on a careful list I had prepared. I realized I needed to prepare certain meals early because we could lose electrical power. I knew we needed a lot of purified water available to drink and we needed to ensure we had certain paper products, cleaning products, and iced green tea and good snacks so we could endure a lengthy storm. I made sure we were making plenty of ice cubes and froze "ice blocks" that would be better able to keep some foods we might have to move to our coolers if we lost power so we would not lose our most important meals. We made sure we had sufficient batteries for certain equipment we would need to use if we lost power for an extensive period as had happened when past hurricanes had come through our area. I made sure all our laundry was washed and the house was cleaned because, based on my past experiences, I wanted to make sure our home would be comfortable if we experienced a bad storm and lost power for an extended time. It was time to listen to "Let it Be" and "Hey Jude" by the Beatles. We were fortunate that we were not hit badly by the hurricane, but The Bahamas suffered in a horrible way. Maybe it is time to listen to "Yellow Submarine" by the Beatles.

I read a lot while we waited to see if the hurricane was going to arrive in Palm Beach County, Florida. I read many magazine articles and thought about my experiences in the last couple of years. Now, I realized you did not have to be a police officer or military officer to be a victim of post-traumatic stress disorder ("PTSD"). I was a victim. Additional reading about PTSD revealed to me that PTSD tended to cause many problems in addition to risk of suicide. Including health problems like heart disease and cancer! Oh my God! I thought I had suffered from PTSD for quite a time before I was diagnosed with cancer in June 2001. Once the storm passed, I searched for a psychologist to consult and made an appointment as soon as possible.

Recently I told my psychologist that I had at least twelve different traumatic events in recent years. (This was far worse than the event when my attacker at my mother's home beat me up and threatened to kill me!) These continuous threats, attacks, and fears is what made my post-traumatic stress disorder ("PTSD") so bad and difficult to heal. Time for a prayer by St. Francis of Assisi: "Lord, make me an instrument of your Life, Love, and Peace..." All of the traumatic events caused my continuing cancer fears—a "side effect of PTSD is cancer, among other significant health problems that are difficult to treat and heal." Each traumatic event I had experienced piled up into a mental mountain for me until I finally found a way to get relief! In the scriptures, the Book of John says: "Ask and you shall receive..." I did. Don called me Dr. C., again. (AAD—Almost a Doctor). The scripture says: "God helps those who help themselves..." "Amen. Thank you, thank you, thank you, God..."

It is well recognized that your brain acts to help you survive. BUT YOU MUST TAKE PROPER ACTION TO THRIVE! Pleasant music, prayers and faith in God can help you survive AND thrive. Listen to "Sundown" by Gordon Lightfoot.

THE END.

Appendix A:

A LIST OF MUSIC REFERENCED FOR YOUR MUSICAL EN-JOYMENT.
FROM MY TOP ONE HUNDRED SONGS
List of Music Referenced in This Book:
5   "Jesus Christ Superstar" from a Broadway Show
6   "Long and Winding Road" by the Beatles
7   "Under Pressure" by Queen
8   "Our House" by Crosby, Stills, Nash and Young
9   "Danny Boy" by the Irish Tenors
10   "With a Little Help From My Friends," by Joe Cocker
11   "Truckin'" by the Grateful Dead
12   "Shake Your Bootie" By K.C. and the Sunshine Band
13   "Yesterday," by the Beatles
14   "Do Not Let Me Down," by the Beatles
15   "Matchmaker" from the movie: *Fiddler on the Roof*, composed by John Williams
16   "Touch of Grey," by the Grateful Dead
17   "I Was Born to Love You," by Queen
18   "American Pie," by Don McLean
19   "As Time Goes By" from the movie *Casablanca*
20   "Tears in Heaven" by Eric Clapton
21   "I Will Survive," by Gloria Gaynor
22   "And So, It Goes" by Billy Joel
23   "Marianne" by Stephen Stills
24   "Ave Maria," sung by Josh Groban and available on Amazon Music (unlimited).
25   *Schindler's List*,
26   "Rocket Man" by Elton John
27   "Irish Lullaby" by the Three Irish Tenors
28   "Earth Angel" by the Penguins

29 "I Go to Extremes" by Billy Joel
30 "Who Wants to Live Forever?" by Queen
31 "C'mon Marianne" by Frankie Valli and the Four Seasons
32 "Eleanor Rigby" by the Beatles
33 "Don't Let the Sun Go Down on Me" by Elton John
34 "Dance with My Father Again" by Byron Lee
35 "Landslide" by Fleetwood MAC
36 "Sargent Pepper's Lonely-Hearts Club Band" by the Beatles
37 "Imagine" by the Beatles
38 "Irish Songs of Rebellion" by the Clancy Brothers
39 "A New York State of Mind" by Billy Joel
40 "Marianne" by Terry Gilkyson and the Easy Riders
41 "He Needed Me" by Anne Murray
42 "Stairway to Heaven" by Led Zeppelin
43 "The Sounds of Silence" by Simon & Garfunkel
44 "Music for the Soul" by Thomas Moore
45 "You May Be Right" by Billy Joel
46 "Good-Bye to Yellow Brook Road" by Elton John
47 "Live and Let Die" by Paul McCartney
48 "Friend of the Devil" by the Grateful Dead
49 "Bohemian Rhapsody" by Queen
50 "Let It Be" by the Beatles
51 "Piano Man" by Billy Joel
52 "Hey Jude" by the Beatles
53 "Rocket Man" by Elton John
54 "Rich Girl" by Daryl Hall and John Oates
55 "Impossible Dream" from the play/movie *Man of La Mancha*
56 "Feelings" by Morris Albert
57 "Take a Walk on the Wild Side" by Lou Reed
58 "Life is a Beach" by the Capitol Steps
59 I Feel the Earth Move Under My Feet" by Carole King
60 "Crocodile Rock" by Elton John
61 "Dream On" by Aerosmith
62 "Helpless" by Simon & Garfunkel
63 "Leaving on a Jet Plane" by Peter, Paul, and Mary

64 "Help" by the Beatles
65 "Thinking Is the Best Way to Travel" and "Tuesday Afternoon" by the Moody Blues
66 "Cecilia" by Simon & Garfunkel
67 "My Sweet Lord" by George Harrison of the Beatles
68 "Your Song" by Elton John
69 "Ode to Joy" by Beethoven
70 "Scenes from an Italian Restaurant" by Billy Joel
71 "Danny Boy," "Sweet Sixteen," "Love's Old Sweet Song," "When Irish Eyes Are Smiling," "The Town I Loved So Well" by the Three Irish Tenors (five different songs)
72 "We Are the Champions" by Queen
73 "Annie's Song" by John Denver
74 "It's a Wild World" by Cat Stevens
75 "Time in a Bottle" by Jim Croce
76 "Hard-Headed Woman" by Cat Stevens
77 "I Am a Rock" by Simon & Garfunkel
78 "Will You Go Lassie Go?" By the Irish Tenors
79 "Nearer My God to Thee" by the Irish Tenors
80 "Amazing Grace" by Women of Ireland from Celtic Airs CD
81 "You Are So Beautiful" by Joe Cocker
82 "The Impossible Dream" sung by Ronan Tynan, an Irish Tenor
83 "Only the Good Die Young" by Billy Joel
84 "I Can't Keep It In" by Cat Stevens
85 "Just the Way You Are" by Billy Joel
86 "She's Got a Way by Billy Joel
87 "Moving Out" by Billy Joel
88 "The Night Is Still Young" by Billy Joel
89 "Big Shot" by Billy Joel
90 "She's Always A Woman" by Billy Joel
91 "Peace Train" by Cat Stevens
92 "My Way" by Frank Sinatra
93 "Escape" by Rupert Holmes (the Pina Colada Song)
94 "Happy Birthday, Baby" by the Tune Weavers
95 "Uptown Girl" by Billy Joel

96 "Moving Out" by Billy Joel
97 "Bridge Over Troubled Water" by Simon & Garfunkel
98 "My Life" by Billy Joel
99 "Let It Be," Hey Jude, and Yellow Submarine by the Beatles
100 "Sundown" by Gordon Lightfoot
101 "Everybody Has a Dream" by Billy Joel
102 A total of 102 songs are listed above.

Appendix B:

PLEASE LOOK UP THE FOLLOWING BOOK TITLES AND ARTICLES WITH INFORMATION AND RESOURCES AND TIPS TO AVOID CHRONIC ILLNESSES OR TREAT THE ROOT CAUSES, INCLUDING TIPS TO AVOID OR OVER-COME CANCER.

Books AND articles to help identify methods to overcome chronic Illnesses and learn how to be an effective advocate for your health:

The Calcium Lie (Calcium Lie II), by Ralph Thompson, MD, and Kathleen Barnes

Protein Equals Pain (Pain Secrets You Won't Hear, From Your Doctor) How to Eliminate the "Joint Pain Protein" and Get Lasting Relief Without Prescription Drugs, Jesse Cannone, CFT, MFT, CPRS

ARTICLE: "How unprocessed trauma is stored in the Body," *Bio Beats.*

MAYO CLINIC BOOK OF HOME REMEDIES, SECOND EDITION, "What to do for the Most Common Health Problems." Cindy Kermott, MD, MPH, and Martha P. Millman, MD, MPH.

The Brain's Way of Healing, New York Times Best Seller, *Remarkable Discoveries and Recoveries from the Frontier of Neuroplasticity,* Norman Doidge, MD, Author of *The Brain that Changes Itself.*

Take Control of Your Life, Rescue Yourself and Live the Life You Deserve, J. Paul Nadeau.

Dance on Your Doctor's Grave! How to be healthy and active at age 100—by going against the conventional medical advice. Frank Shallenberger, MD, Author of *Bursting with Energy.*

Peace Is Every Step, The Path of Mindfulness in Everyday Life. The San Francisco Chronicle wrote: "Lucidity adapts...ancient Buddhist teachings to...modern problems...Terrific...Hypnotic...Subtle and extremely effective."

How to Talk so Your Husband Will Listen, Rick Johnson.

The Plant Paradox, New York Times Best Seller, *The Hidden Dangers in "Healthy" Foods that Cause Disease and Weight Gain*, Steven R. Gundry, MD.

Dr. Gundry's Diet Evolution Turn Off the Genes that are Killing You and Your Waistline, Features: 70 recipes, sample menus, and memory tricks to keep you on track.

The Plant Paradox Cookbook, New York Times Best Seller, Steven R. Gundry, MD.

How to Get Along with Difficult People, Florence Littauer.

Spontaneous Healing by Andrew Weil, M.D.

After Cancer, A Guide To Your New Life by Wendy Schlessel Harpham, MD.

Finding God in the Plague, New York Times Best Seller, Mike Evans.

Positive Thinking by Norman Vincent Peale.

Age Healthier Live Healthier, Avoiding Over-Medication through Natural Hormone Balance by Dr. Gary Donovitz

OTHER BOOKS FOR ENJOYMENT:

The Lincoln Myth, a novel. Steve Berry, *New York Times* Bestselling Author of the King's Deception.

Abraham Lincoln, Quotes, Quips, AND Speeches, Gordon Leidner, Editor.

Tuesdays with Morrie, An old man, a young man, and life's greatest lesson, Mitch Albom.

So, You Think You Are Irish, Margaret Kelleher.

How the Irish Saved Civilization, The Untold Story of Ireland's Heroic Role from the Fall of Rome to Rise of Medieval Europe, Thomas Cahill, "Charming and Poetic…an entirely engaging, delectable voyage into the distant past, a small treasure." Quote from Richard Bernstein, *The New York Times*.

The Gifts of the Jews. How a Tribe of Desert Nomads Changed the Way Everyone Thinks and Feels, Thomas Cahill, Author of How the Irish Saved Civilization.

Irish Wit & Wisdom, Gil Books of Dublin Ireland.

Saving Lives Saving Dignity, an Amazon Best Seller published in 2020 (includes guidance about "End of Life" procedures). And the authors are Alan Molk, MD, and Robert A. Shapiro, MD (ER physicians in Phoenix, Arizona).

You can also search for articles/newsletter publications and subscribe to regular updated information by the following organizations to improve your health and wellness:

Harvard Women's Health Watch

Harvard Heart Letter

Harvard Health Letter

Cleveland Clinic Heart Advisor

Massachusetts General Hospital, "Mind, Mood & Memory"

Appendix C

TIPS FOR HEALTH AND WELLNESS

Dietary suggestions to avoid cancer (from American Cancer Society):

Avoid Alcohol

Do not use tobacco products

Maintain healthy weight

Get plenty of physical activity

Eat plenty of fruits and vegetables

Avoid mid-day sunshine and use hat, shirt to protect skin (You may need to cut the amount of sunscreen you use if it has dangerous metal ingredients.)

Get recommended cancer screening tests.

Call 1-800-227-2345 or visit cancer.org for more information.

My suggestions:

Avoid fruits, vegetable, soy products produced in the US UNLESS they are organically grown to avoid consumption of harmful "roundup" used to grow US crops. European products are better because the Europeans banned use of roundup years ago.

Avoid sugar during cancer treatment to keep from growing cancer cells.

Develop good sleeping habits to keep immune system high to avoid growth of cancer cells.

Listen to calming and relaxing music daily to help kill cancer cells.

The Mayo Clinic announced a new treatment for cancer to substitute for chemotherapy that has bad side effects:

The new treatment is based on a certain kind of laser treatment so you do not have to pump your body full of harmful medicines/chemicals, but the new treatment is only available at select locations.

Avoid deep depression:

Try getting electro convulsive therapy (ECT) to avoid excess use of antidepressants.

Pursue psychological therapy.

Keep a regular written journal to alleviate concerns that could lead to depression or other problems.

PURSUE REMEDIES FOR POST-TRAUMATIC STRESS DISORDER (PTSD):

PTSD can increase anxiety, depression, anger, frustration, sleep disorder, and can increase risk of suicide and cancer.

If you "self-medicate" with alcohol, be careful not to drink excessively and get good psychological therapy.

Try plant-based, natural hormone replacement therapy as it decreases the above problems (regular replacement therapy can lead to cancer).

Sleep tips:

"Best Sleep" is "NO PILLS" for sleep. Pills do not cure the root cause of sleep problems. The pills can cause sleep disturbance, especially when you take them on a long-term basis. There are new studies available to treat root causes of a sleep disorder without Big Pharma drugs. You may need to have a test done to see if you have sleep apnea and find out the best treatment for that problem, after considering these comments/tips.

Listen to music to prepare for sleep and begin relaxation about an hour before bedtime.

Avoid working on computer and watching TV soon before bedtime to keep "blue rays" from contributing to insomnia.

Try to use lavender oil and lotion before bedtime to increase relaxation and sleepiness.

Try consuming "Sleepy Time" herbal tea as well.

Meditate prior to bedtime to help make you sleepy.

Consume liquid melatonin , which is more easily absorbed, and/or melatonin in "gummy" form early before bedtime to allow your body to properly absorb it, in order to increase the length of your sleep through the night.